PRAISE FOR
Queer Expressions

"Wednesdae is able to weave together expressive arts, somatic awareness, and trauma-informed care in a way that is both deeply personal and widely resonant. Their work honors the complexities of queer embodiment while offering concrete, compassionate pathways for healing. . . . This is not a book about technique for its own sake—it's a deeply considered, liberatory framework where art becomes a tool for survival, self-expression, and transformation.

Wednesdae's vibrant soul and compassion shine through in their writing, which holds space for all bodies, identities, and stories with gentleness and empowerment. I believe this will be a vital resource for clinicians, educators, and anyone invested in creating more compassionate, just, and creative possibilities for body-based and expressive arts healing."

—JACKIE ARMSTRONG, MA (she/they), associate educator, visitor research and experience at The Museum of Modern Art

"Wednesdae delivers a master class in the art of healing. They fuse expressive and somatic therapies with precision, compassion, and heart, showing how creativity can transform pain into power. Their writing moves, teaches, and inspires in equal measure—inviting readers to pick up the brush, the pen, or the dance step and reclaim their own narratives. This book doesn't just inform; it ignites."

—MONIKA OSTROFF, LICSW, CEDS-S (she/they), executive director of MEDA (Multi-Service Eating Disorder Association)

"This book offers a clear, incisive integration of expressive arts and body-based therapies for work with queer and trans communities, making creative processes with LGBTQIA+ clients accessible to both new and seasoned practitioners. Themes of liberation, harm reduction, anti-oppressive practice, agency, and social justice are treated with rigor and heart. Through vivid client narratives, Wednesdae bridges theory and practice and reminds us that arts therapies must ultimately make our clients' lives more livable, hospitable, and joyful. A timely, essential read for anyone studying or supporting LGBTQIA+ lives through creative therapeutic practice."

—ZACHARY D. VAN DEN BERG, MA, ATR-BC, LPC, author and editor of *Queer Worldmaking in Art Therapy*, art therapist and counselor, and president and founder of the Coalition for Queer Creative Arts Therapies, Inc.

QUEER EXPRESSIONS

QUEER EXPRESSIONS

EXPRESSIVE ART AND SOMATIC THERAPY PRACTICES FOR HEALING BODY TRAUMA

WEDNESDAE REIM IFRACH
REAT, ATR-BC, CLAT

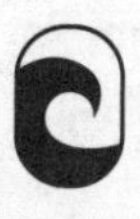

North Atlantic Books
Huichin, unceded Ohlone land
Berkeley, California

North Atlantic Books
Huichin, unceded Ohlone land
2526 Martin Luther King Jr Way
Berkeley, CA 94704 USA
www.northatlanticbooks.com

Cover art © Kupalina via Getty Images
Cover design by Jasmine Hromjak
Book design by Happenstance Type-O-Rama

Printed in the United States of America

Queer Expressions: Expressive Art and Somatic Therapy Practices for Healing Body Trauma is sponsored and published by North Atlantic Books, an educational nonprofit that collaborates with partners to develop cross-cultural perspectives; nurture holistic views of art, science, the humanities, and healing; and seed personal and global transformation by publishing work on the relationship of body, spirit, and nature.

North Atlantic Books's publications are distributed to the US trade and internationally by Penguin Random House Publisher Services. For further information, visit our website at www.northatlanticbooks.com.

The authorized representative in the EU for product safety and compliance is Eucomply OÜ, Pärnu mnt 139b-14, 11317 Tallinn, Estonia, hello@eucompliancepartner.com, +33757690241.

Library of Congress Cataloging-in-Publication Data

Names: Ifrach, Wednesdae Reim author | Wooding, Megan photographer
Title: Queer expressions : expressive art and somatic therapy practices for healing body trauma / Wednesdae Reim Ifrach, REAT, CLAT ; photography by Megan Wooding.
Description: Berkeley, CA : North Atlantic Books, [2026] | Includes bibliographical references and index. | Summary: "A guide to healing body trauma through embodiment and creativity for queer, trans, and gender-expansive readers"— Provided by publisher.
Identifiers: LCCN 2026001053 (print) | LCCN 2026001054 (ebook) | ISBN 9798889843191 trade paperback | ISBN 9798889843207 ebook
Subjects: LCSH: Psychic trauma | Healing—Psychological aspects | Sexual minorities—Psychology
Classification: LCC BF175.5.P75 I38 2026 (print) | LCC BF175.5.P75 (ebook)
LC record available at https://lccn.loc.gov/2026001053
LC ebook record available at https://lccn.loc.gov/2026001054

1 2 3 4 5 6 7 8 9 KPC 31 30 29 28 27 26

To my nephew Felix, who shows me each day that
love, belonging, and celebration are birthrights.
Your spirit reminds me that wonder and
creativity hold the power to heal.

Contents

Acknowledgments

To my partner, Ron, thank you for your unwavering faith in me, for standing by my side each time I say yes to work that is both challenging and beautiful. Thank you for the long car rides, '90s music, horror movies on repeat, for our shared love of art and art therapy, and for being the kind of partner who makes the world a better place.

To my parents, thank you for believing in me even when things didn't make sense, were difficult, or got complicated. Thank you for supporting dreams that may have seemed impossible or wild.

To my brother Adam, my sister-in-law Anne, and my nephew Felix, thank you for the group chats with inappropriate memes, bedtime stories, *It's Always Sunny*, and the infamous pizza debates. Our humor taught me that grounding is more than breathing; it is living in the present.

To all my friends, especially Kayti, my chosen family, thank you for holding space, for seeing me, loving me, believing in me, and fighting for me.

To my oldest friend Nicky (Annick), thank you for being in my corner for most of our lives. We have survived more than can fit in a few sentences. Thank you for being my family, and for knowing we always come home.

To my therapist, thank you for over ten years of holding space, helping me grow and navigate the world. You have made my world a better place to be in.

To every art therapist and expressive art therapist in my life, to my mentors, supervisors, professors, and colleagues, thank you. A small piece of each of you and your guidance found its way into these pages.

To my clients, past, present, and future, none of this would be possible without your trust. Thank you for allowing me to guide you, for giving the feedback that helped me grow as a therapist and a person, and for proving that growth is uncomfortable, therapists are human, and we are always in parallel process.

To the Queer community, we are here, we have always been here, and we will always be here. Our bodies and hearts deserve space to be seen, witnessed, and heard so that we can thrive. Never stop healing. Never stop loving. Never stop, because we are, and always will be, here.

Foreword

As a Queer artist, art therapist, expressive art therapist, and somatic therapist, I often say that this work is what saved me. That's the transformative power of art and somatics. As a person in recovery from an eating disorder and complex trauma, my relationship with my body has been shaped by both violence and resilience, by systems that tried to erase me, and by communities that insisted I was worth saving. This book grows from that lineage: from the messy, tender, and courageous work of making a home in my skin.

My earliest relationship to creativity was not about beauty but about survival. Creativity was a tool that empowered me to navigate the complexities of my identity. I drew before I could write sentences. I moved my body in strange, unselfconscious shapes before I knew what dance was "supposed" to look like. In my sketchbooks, I could explore the feelings that felt too dangerous to name. In my poems, I could wrap truths in metaphor so they might be spoken without being stolen. I didn't yet know I was Queer, but I knew what it was to live with secrets. My art was my first and most loyal witness.

As I got older, I also learned that my body was a site of other people's judgments, something to be evaluated, disciplined, and fixed. I learned to shrink myself, not only in size but in voice and gesture. My eating disorder was, in some ways, an attempt to gain control in a world that felt unsafe. Recovery, for me, was not simply about eating differently. It was about *being* different. And for that, I needed both creativity and embodiment.

Queer communities have always known how to create alchemy from the raw material of our survival. The dance floor at a gay bar. The catwalk at a drag ball. The swell of voices chanting at a protest. These are not just sites of entertainment or politics; they are somatic laboratories, places where bodies learn new rhythms of safety and expression.

Ballroom culture, for example, emerged as a Black and Latino underground subculture, creating spaces where people estranged from their families could find chosen kinship. To vogue is to tell a story with the body: sharp angles of arms, liquid rolls of hips, sudden freezes, bursts of release. It is an aesthetic and somatic strategy, as well as discipline and liberation, in the same breath. These embodied practices are not separate from healing; they *are* healing, especially for bodies told they do not belong.

Research affirms what these cultural practices have always known: The body is both a repository of trauma and a site of potential repair. Somatic therapies work with the nervous system to help people renegotiate threat responses, release stored tension, and cultivate a sense of safety. Expressive art therapies engage sensory, kinesthetic, and symbolic modes of communication that bypass the limitations of verbal processing. When combined, these approaches invite a dialogue between the body and imagination, allowing sensation, image, and movement to become fluent languages of healing. For Queer clients, many of whom have been silenced, shamed, or pathologized in traditional therapeutic settings, the combination of somatic and expressive arts practices vitally disrupts that silence; it offers a way to speak without words, to listen without judgment, to reclaim the body as subject rather than object.

I have seen, in my own life and my work with clients, what happens when art and somatics meet. I have seen the trans man who could not look at his reflection paint his silhouette in colors he called "future." I have seen the non-binary teen who hid their voice in public sing for the first time in a therapy session, trembling but unbroken. I have seen a survivor of sexual violence reclaim the rhythm of their breath through slow, mindful movement, and with it, the possibility of pleasure.

These moments matter because they are more than therapeutic progress; they are political acts. To feel safe in a Queer body is to resist centuries of messages that say you should not. To create from that body is to declare it worthy of attention, of beauty, of space.

Of course, Queer embodiment is not a singular experience. It's a complex interplay of various identities and experiences. Intersectionality reminds us that race, class, gender identity, sexuality, disability, and immigration status shape how bodies move through the world and how safe they feel doing so. A Black trans woman navigating public space carries a different set of somatic adaptations than a white cisgender lesbian; a disabled Queer immigrant may find liberation not in dance but in digital collage or breath-based practices. Healing work must be expansive enough to hold these differences without erasing them, validating the unique experiences of each individual.

This book approaches body trauma through four interconnected frameworks: expressive arts, somatic therapy, body liberation, and harm reduction. Body liberation is a concept that challenges societal beauty norms and the idea that worth is tied to physical appearance. Harm reduction meets people where they are, without imposing a single, "right" path. In combination, they allow therapy to become a co-created, consent-based practice grounded in justice as much as in care.

This book is for anyone who has carried their story in the curve of their spine, in the shallowness of their breath, in the way they shrink or take up space. For the Queer kid sketching their truth in the margins. For the trans adult who feels safest in motion. For the therapist willing to hold complexity without rushing toward resolution.

Queer healing, as I have come to know it, is not simply about repairing what has been broken. It is about generating wholly new worlds, selves, and relationships expansive enough to contain our multiplicity. Liberation is not merely the absence of harm; it is the ongoing presence of joy, agency, and creative possibility. That is the vision at the heart of *Queer Expressions*, that we deserve not only to survive, but to create lives and bodies that are unapologetically our own.

1

Queer Bodies' Narratives

Expressive art therapy is a form of psychotherapy that utilizes creative processes, including drawing, painting, sculpting, movement, music, drama, and writing, as vehicles for clients' self-expression, emotional exploration, introspection, coping, and healing. This form of therapy, grounded in psychotherapy, psychology, and counseling, focuses on four core principles: nonverbal communication; the therapeutic process being more important than the art product; holistic integration of mind, body, and spirit; and client-centered strength-based approaches.[1] Clients are given the space to discover their emotional experiences that lie beneath conscious awareness, experiences too complex to put into words. By engaging in art-making, clients can express embodied or preverbal material in a symbolic, sensory, and metaphorical language.[2] Expressive art therapy attends to mind, body, and spirit. It acknowledges that psychological distress often manifests somatically, and that creative activity can promote embodiment, regulation, and a sense of agency.

This work honors clients as experts in their own lives. As the therapist, I provide a supportive, nonjudgmental environment that nurtures autonomy, resilience, and self-efficacy. Through expressive art therapy, clients can focus on trauma processing in a contained, gradual way, approaching traumatic memories through metaphors and at a safe distance. The therapy also enables emotional regulation by supporting clients in engaging in rhythmic or sensory activities, which can help down-regulate hyperarousal or up-regulate hypoarousal.[3] Neurodiverse clients can experience support through an alternative mode of communication, which is particularly effective for clients with language challenges, autism spectrum diagnoses, or intellectual disabilities. Through identity and self-esteem work, clients can create tangible artifacts to support exploration of their strengths, values, and evolving self-concept, which is especially powerful for marginalized populations.

Expressive art therapy naturally pairs with somatic therapy as a way to provide a holistic experience. Somatic therapy is a body-based form of psychotherapy that emphasizes the connection between mind and body in the healing of trauma, stress, and emotional dysregulation. By bringing mindful awareness to bodily sensations, movement patterns, posture, and breath, somatic therapy aims to release stored tension and trauma that may be held below conscious awareness. Somatic therapies integrate both body and mind to address psychological distress, which often manifests physically: tight muscles, shallow breathing, and chronic pain. Somatic therapy posits that by attending to bodily signals, clients can access and process emotional or traumatic material that verbal talk alone may not reach. When clinically appropriate, cultivating a compassionate and curious attention to internal sensations can support interoceptive awareness, which helps clients differentiate between overwhelming reactivity and tolerable arousal, and build the capacity to stay "in the window of functionality." It also allows for regulation before processing, rather than diving straight into traumatic memories or verbalization that can re-traumatize a client.[4]

In my work, the most common form of expressive art therapy I employ is a combination of somatic breathwork and movement, along with traditional visual arts. This may look like some deep grounding breaths and the client setting an intention for the session, such as "I'd like clarity on how to cope with trauma symptoms developing in my body." From there, we discuss their boundaries and what feels safe and authentic to them, based on our therapeutic relationship and the length of treatment. Then I may ask the client if they can do a movement or two that could represent the way they think their body might feel if they didn't feel their trauma in their body. We might discuss how that movement felt in their bodies: "Did something feel weighted versus light, fluid versus bumpy, relieving versus activating?" From there, I ask the client to label colors and shapes that correlate with what they think it would feel like if they felt empowered in managing their symptoms. This then translates to creating a painting, collage, drawing, or visual representation of that, and using it to evoke a sense of relief and empowerment during the session. In this way, the piece serves as a space to hold on to hope and to reorient oneself.

Somatic therapy emphasizes first orienting and then down-regulating the nervous system through grounding exercises, breathwork, and gentle movement, which creates a safe environment for deeper work. Much like expressive art therapy, somatic therapy supports working through trauma by allowing gradual, titrated engagement with traumatic material, reducing the risk of re-traumatization. It also supports clients in noticing early somatic signs of panic and anxiety and downshifting physiologically before a crisis.[5] Somatic therapy and expressive art therapy allow bodies, especially marginalized bodies, to be able to embody their stories.

Bodily Narratives

Narratives or stories documenting our cultures, experiences, and evolutions are integral to the human experience. Therapists have come to understand the essential role that personal, familial, cultural, and global narratives play in self-concept, identity formation, personal growth, and development. Through the multiple layers a narrative holds, clients begin to unravel the essence of who a person is, who they are, and what they view as crucial to their story. Therapists can support clients in unraveling their narrative threads and extracting the pieces that feel meaningful to the client. We can see the complete narrative while honoring their most important threads. As therapists, we need to understand how these narratives shape people and create the schema through which they see the world.[6] Without narratives, people lose parts of themselves. It could be a disconnect from a personal event, a family story passed down for generations, or stories from culture, ethnicity, or other identities. Even when someone cannot remember a story, the body holds on to narratives. These narratives can be seen through sociocultural concepts supported by epigenetic theories on intergenerational trauma and how generations of trauma can shift DNA long term.[7] This means that bodies tell a story comprised of multiple narratives of a complex and complicated existence. The more marginalized a body, the more complex the narrative and the body's experience in the world.

Queer narratives hold personal, familial, romantic, sexual, political, national, and global areas of functioning. Understanding the intersections of these narratives and how our bodies encapsulate them can be an illuminating experience. Clients can discover ways to express these narratives, leading to a meaningful release and a sense of liberation that deepens their connection to their body and identities. Queer narratives come with a complex cultural history. This is a narrative each Queer individual carries within them, even if the person is not fully aware of it.[8]

In expanding the exploration of Queer bodies and narratives, it is crucial to consider the clients' stories and how they are constructed, stored, and expressed. Narrative work has evolved to acknowledge that language, memory, and the body are part of it. Storytelling is more than a cognitive experience; it is an embodied practice that engages neural, physiological, and emotional systems. Each person comes into Queerness differently. For some it is a painful journey; for others it can be a positive and affirming experience. Examining our narratives is a complicated experience. Often, Queer therapists sit in the liminal space of constantly reviewing their individual narratives in a parallel process with their clients, and this can be a gift. If we, as therapists, hold similar identities with our clients, especially Queer identities, we need to continuously be aware of our parallel process, transference, countertransference, and biases.[9] Awareness allows us to support the client in examining their personal narrative and moving into a different space and frame of mind. It is no longer a cognitive, verbal space where the person holds a list of traumas and successes, the critical moments that have made an impact. Instead, it is a summation of the experience, where clients can be challenged to list the feelings attached to it and further delve into the body's connection to it: *What has the nervous system held on to? What moments has our autonomic system held on to?*

The autonomic nervous system oversees the fight, flight, freeze, and fawn responses. It is the central system for all our unconscious functions, including breathing, digestion, and heart rate. It plays a crucial role in our responses to trauma. By associating somatic responses with their narratives, our clients can uncover the existential meaning behind them. This process allows them to work through the parts of trauma that remain attached to those experiences.[10] As therapists, our role is to aid in unraveling the client's narrative once they have labeled the parts their nervous system has held on to.

It is important to honor that Queer identities do not exist in isolation. They are intertwined with all parts of the identity, such as race, class, gender, religion, ethnicity, ability status, sexuality, and culture. The intersectional nature of these identities means multiple sources of oppression and privilege exist simultaneously. Intersectionality, as a framework, asks therapists to recognize that each intersecting identity brings histories, traumas, and strengths that inform the client's understanding of their body, narrative, and the places they can inhabit. Understanding intersectionality is fundamental in therapeutic contexts, where clients may struggle with internalized stigma or conflicting narratives about their worth. When we integrate these multiple narratives, the therapeutic space becomes a place where the validity of each aspect of a client's identity is affirmed, and healing is facilitated. This means attending to recounting stories and the subtle bodily cues that signal internal conflict or resilience.

It is impossible to discuss Queer body narratives without acknowledging the broader cultural and political landscape. Queer identities continue to be contested and politicized. The public discourse surrounding Queer issues often oscillates between celebration and vilification, reflecting broader societal tensions about gender, sexuality, and power. For many Queer individuals, the act of coming out and living authentically is both a personal liberation and a political statement. The intersection of personal and political is vividly illustrated in how bodies can be read as texts, sites where the marks of oppression, resistance, and survival are inscribed. The shared trauma of discrimination, harassment, and systemic violence reinforces a collective memory that is both painful and empowering. By acknowledging these political dimensions in therapy, clients can begin contextualizing their experiences within a larger sociopolitical framework, recognizing that their personal stories are part of a broader narrative of struggle and resistance.

In the therapeutic setting, this recognition can be empowering. Clients who see their experiences as part of a more significant movement often feel a sense of solidarity and validation. They are reminded that their struggles are not isolated incidents but connected to a long history of resilience and activism. This perspective can transform the narrative, reframing the client's story as empowerment, where the body's responses, though shaped by trauma, reflect strength, creativity, and a capacity for transformation.

The concept of embodied memory is central to understanding the somatic dimension of trauma. Embodied memory refers to the idea that traumatic experiences are stored in the mind and imprinted in the body. When a traumatic event occurs, particularly during critical developmental periods, the body "remembers" it through sensory and physiological reactions ranging from rapid heart rate to subtle posture shifts or muscle tension. For Queer individuals whose early encounters with trauma are linked with experiences of rejection or abuse, these bodily imprints become intertwined with the narrative of their identity.

Epigenetic research further reinforces this perspective by suggesting that trauma can lead to biological changes that are passed down through generations. The transmission of these biological markers means that the effects of trauma can persist long after the original event, influencing how subsequent generations experience stress and resilience. Such research underlines the importance of addressing both the psychological and the somatic dimensions of trauma in therapeutic work. By understanding that the body holds stories that may not be accessible to conscious memory, therapists can validate experiences that clients might otherwise struggle to articulate.[11]

Storytelling is more than merely recounting past events; it is an active process of re-creation and meaning-making. Within the therapeutic context, storytelling allows clients to reframe their experiences by integrating their histories' painful and empowering aspects. This re-narration is a transformative process that can alter how individuals see themselves and their place in the world. For example, when a client reconfigures a narrative of loss or betrayal into one of survival and resilience, storytelling becomes a vehicle for reclaiming agency over their life. This is particularly poignant for Queer individuals, who may have had their authentic selves invalidated by dominant cultural narratives. Crafting one's narrative can involve several therapeutic techniques, including journaling, guided imagery, role-playing, and digital storytelling. Each method invites clients to explore their past experiences while envisioning alternative futures. By engaging in these creative acts, clients may begin dismantling the rigid frameworks imposed by societal expectations and instead forge narratives that celebrate the fluidity and multiplicity of their identities.

Furthermore, incorporating cultural narratives and stories that speak to shared histories, mythologies, and traditions can offer clients a sense of belonging and continuity. For many Queer individuals, reconnecting with or reclaiming cultural narratives that have been marginalized or suppressed can be an act of defiance against dominant discourses that have historically devalued their existence. By weaving these collective narratives into their personal story, clients not only affirm their individual experiences but also participate in creating a broader cultural tapestry that challenges systemic oppression. The body is not merely a vessel for carrying genetic material but a dynamic repository of experience. Every sensation, every movement, and every reaction is imbued with the memories of past encounters. In trauma theory, the body is often described as a "holding space" for memories that the mind may not consciously recall. Somatic memory strongly affects how individuals experience and respond to their current stressors. For Queer individuals, whose bodies may have been the site of repeated assaults, whether physical, emotional, or systemic, the body holds a complex matrix of responses that are both protective and, at times, limiting.

The interplay between the autonomic nervous system and embodied memory is particularly significant in therapeutic work. Techniques focusing on body awareness, such as mindfulness, yoga, and somatic experiencing, enable clients to access and modulate these deep-seated responses. For instance, by learning to recognize subtle changes in muscle tension or shifts in breathing patterns, clients can begin to identify when their body is reliving past trauma. This increased awareness is a critical first step in creating new patterns of response that are more adaptive and grounded in the present moment.

In practical terms, therapists might integrate body-based interventions into their sessions to help clients reconnect with their physical sensations in a safe and structured way. Through practices such as progressive muscle relaxation or guided body scans, clients can learn to differentiate between the echoes of past trauma and their current bodily experience. Over time, this enhanced somatic awareness can empower clients to reclaim control over their reactions, opening up new healing and integration pathways.

The concept of intersectionality provides a vital framework for understanding how multiple forms of identity and oppression interact to shape the lived experience of Queer individuals.[12] For example, while a white gay man might navigate specific social spaces with relative ease, a Black transgender person may face compounded barriers due to both racism and transphobia. Equally, the same white gay man might be at a corporate event and experience homophobia through microaggressions such as slurs for Queer people. The same Black transgender woman may participate in a Black-led community event where they may not experience racism but may experience transphobia. Similarly, a gay Black man may experience homophobia at the same community event.

Within the therapeutic space, intersectionality calls for an attuned sensitivity to how various aspects of a client's identity interact and impact their narrative, rather than offering a one-size-fits-all approach to healing.

This might involve creating spaces where clients can explore how cultural traditions, family histories, and social expectations intersect with their Queer identity. Recognizing this multiplicity is essential in tailoring therapeutic approaches that honor the full spectrum of a client's experiences.

Moreover, intersectional analysis in therapy can guide therapists to address systemic issues contributing to a client's distress. It is not enough to focus solely on the individual; the broader social and political context must also be acknowledged. This may lead to integrating social justice work into the therapeutic process, whether by facilitating community connections, advocating for policy changes, or simply validating the client's experiences as part of a larger narrative of resistance and resilience. Integrating the insights of embodied narrative theory into clinical practice has given rise to some innovative therapeutic interventions that combine traditional narrative techniques with somatic practices to facilitate psychological and physical healing. For example, somatic experiencing is a modality that focuses on releasing the energy held within the body due to traumatic experiences. By encouraging clients to notice and name the sensations they feel (tension, warmth, a racing heartbeat), therapists help them access and process memories that might otherwise remain locked away in the body.

Similarly, expressive art therapy invites clients to externalize their internal experiences through creative expression. Painting, collage, or digital storytelling offers a nonverbal means of communicating complex emotions and memories. For Queer individuals, art therapy can be particularly transformative, as it allows for the creation of a visual language that transcends the limitations of traditional discourse. In doing so, it empowers clients to reclaim narratives silenced or distorted by societal pressures.

Movement-based therapies, such as dance and mindful movement, further enhance the integration of embodied experience. These practices recognize that the body is not a passive recipient of trauma but an active participant in the healing process. By engaging in free-form movement or structured practices like yoga, clients can begin to reshape their relationship with their body. They learn to experience their physicality as a source of strength and creativity rather than as a repository of pain. This reorientation facilitates the release of traumatic energy and fosters a renewed connection to one's embodied self.

Therapists may also utilize guided imagery techniques that encourage clients to envision their body as a site of healing and transformation. In these exercises, the client might be guided to imagine a place of safety within their body, a sanctuary where the wounds of the past can begin to mend. Such imagery can help bridge the gap between conscious narrative and unconscious embodied memory, offering a pathway for integrating disparate aspects of the self.

The work of facilitating embodied narrative healing is deeply relational. For therapists, engaging with clients' stories requires an ongoing commitment to self-reflection and self-care. Many Queer therapists find that their personal histories resonate with those of their clients, creating a shared space of vulnerability and insight. This parallel process, while potentially enriching, also demands careful navigation. Therapists must remain vigilant about their unresolved traumas, biases, and countertransference issues to ensure that the therapeutic space remains centered on the client's needs. Supervision, peer consultation, and personal therapy are indispensable tools for therapists in this field. These supports enable therapists to process their own experiences and emotions, thereby preventing burnout and maintaining the integrity of the therapeutic process.

In addition, engaging in continuous education around topics such as intersectionality, trauma-informed care, and somatic practices helps therapists remain attuned to the evolving needs of their clients. When therapists are deeply connected to their own embodied experiences, they are better positioned to meet clients where they are, both physically and emotionally, and to foster an environment of trust and safety. Empathy, as both a clinical skill and a personal quality, lies at the heart of practical narrative work. Through empathy, therapists can validate their clients' lived experiences, affirming the legitimacy of their stories even when these narratives challenge dominant cultural discourses. In this process, I act as a witness to the client's suffering and co-creator of a narrative emphasizing resilience and hope. By sharing the client's transformation journey, I help reframe trauma as a source of insight rather than a permanent mark of defeat.

The integration of social and political activism into therapeutic narratives represents a powerful frontier in the field of trauma therapy. Many Queer individuals cannot fully realize their personal healing without addressing the systemic forces that contribute to their pain. Recognizing the interplay between personal trauma and societal injustice, therapists can work collaboratively with clients to foster a sense of empowerment that extends beyond the therapy room. One way to achieve this is incorporating community building and collective storytelling into the therapeutic process. Group therapy sessions, community art projects, and public narrative forums allow clients to share their experiences in a supportive environment. This creates a counter-narrative to the dominant discourses of marginalization and oppression. In these settings, the individual narrative is amplified by the voices of others who share similar struggles, transforming isolated pain into a collective force for change.

Therapists can play an active role in advocating for policy reforms and social justice initiatives that impact the Queer community. By staying informed about the political and social issues affecting their clients, therapists can offer guidance on navigating and challenging oppressive systems. This might involve connecting clients with activist organizations, facilitating discussions about community organizing, or simply acknowledging the role of systemic injustice in the client's narrative. When the therapeutic process becomes intertwined with broader movements for social change, it reinforces the idea that healing is both an individual and a collective endeavor. The field of embodied narrative therapy continues to evolve, with ongoing research illuminating new pathways for integrating mind, body, and story. Emerging techniques, such as neurofeedback and sensorimotor psychotherapy, hold promise for deepening our understanding of how the body processes trauma and how these processes can be modified to support healing. These innovations underscore the importance of interdisciplinary collaboration as insights from neuroscience, psychology, and cultural studies converge to create more comprehensive therapy models.

One promising direction is the application of technology to enhance embodied narrative work. Virtual reality, for instance, has been used experimentally to help clients visualize and interact with aspects of their narrative in immersive ways. Such technologies can provide safe, controlled environments where clients confront and reframe traumatic memories, an experiential form of therapy that complements traditional verbal methods. While still in its early stages, a digital tool with embodied narrative techniques represents an exciting frontier that may offer new hope for those who struggle to access their buried memories through conventional approaches. At the same time, the growing recognition of the importance of cultural competence in therapy has led to a more nuanced understanding of how diverse narratives intersect with individual healing. Research into culturally responsive therapeutic practices continues to emphasize the need for therapists to integrate their clients' unique historical and social contexts into the narrative process. For Queer individuals, this means acknowledging not only the personal dimensions of their story but also the collective memory of resistance, survival, and transformation that defines their community.

Narratives are more than mere stories; they are the foundation upon which identities are built and transformed. As the field of psychotherapy moves toward more integrative and culturally informed models of care, the insights gained from embodied narrative work offer a roadmap for addressing the profound challenges of trauma and marginalization. Therapists are not merely facilitators of verbal recounting; they are co-creators of a narrative that holds the potential to transform personal suffering into a source of collective strength and hope. In this transformative process, every memory, every sensation, and every story become a vital thread in the fabric of human resilience, a fabric that, when woven together, can create a tapestry of healing that defies even the most entrenched systems of oppression.

Ultimately, untangling and reweaving our narratives is an ongoing journey that invites us to revisit and reshape our stories as we evolve continuously. For Queer individuals and all those whose dominant cultural narratives have been marginalized, this work is both a personal and a political act. It is an act of reclaiming the body, asserting one's identity, and challenging the forces that seek to silence our voices. As therapists and human beings, we are called to honor these stories, listen deeply, and help transform the raw material of lived experience into a narrative of empowerment, resilience, and hope. In embracing the full complexity of our narratives, we acknowledge that healing is not a linear process but a multifaceted journey that touches every aspect of our being: physical, emotional, cognitive, and spiritual. It is a journey that requires us to be courageous, confront the painful echoes of the past, and envision a future where every voice is heard, every body is celebrated, and every story is valued.

Case Example: Sensory Art for Queer Narrative Exploration

Over the years, I have worked with many Queer clients of all different backgrounds. This client was a white transgender man (he/they) in his late twenties, raised in a middle-class household. He experienced extensive childhood trauma growing up in a violent household, and his extended family often made comments about food, weight, and his body, which became a primary focus. He became acutely aware of his body and developed an eating disorder on top of complex post-traumatic stress disorder (CPTSD). Years later, he realized he was Queer and came out as a transgender man, but because he'd been raised in an environment where he was constantly in fight-or-flight and where trusted adults shamed his body, the idea of being publicly Queer triggered that autonomic response.

In our work together, we examined this narrative and asked, "Where did personal awareness of the body start?" He shared that he could remember being frightened at three years old, not understanding why the adults were scary and loud, why adults were scaring him, and hiding under the bed, feeling his heart pounding. So his somatic narrative, which refers to the bodily sensations and reactions that are part of his narrative, starts with his heart beating at three years old, then a series of events of becoming aware of his body and food. From the ages of twelve to eighteen, he can remember having frequent experiences of feeling dissociated from his body, and he can remember the sensation of his skin crawling when he became grounded in his body. He could even recall the sensation of wanting to run from his family in his body.

When prompted for a parallel narrative of positive sensations, he shared remembering his time with his grandparents, specifically his grandmother. He can remember how her skin would often feel warm, like he was being wrapped in a blanket, and how he would often feel a sense of calm when she was around, like it was easier to breathe and be in his body. Now the client takes all these competing experiences and sees the convergence of the personal and familial narrative and how it lives within the nervous system. Underneath all of this is still the impending Queer narrative that cannot stay buried.[13]

From here, the client could then delve into the romantic and sexual narrative, where the suppressed parts of the Queer-self needed space to be explored. These parts manifest in various ways, denying the true self. However, this is also where the transformative power of art and somatic work comes into play, offering a beacon of hope. In this case, confronting his Queer identity meant facing personal and familial trauma. By examining the somatic attachment to that narrative, he could see the sensation of heart pounding, shortness of breath, flight responses, and tactile aversion as his trauma responses. Simultaneously, there was the experience of the joy of warmth, calm, and feeling blanketed. Embracing these positive experiences is possible by creating art around these flight responses.[14]

The client made a visual artwork encompassing those experiences, incorporating each sensory experience (see Figure 1). In this process, I offered questions that focused on his sensory experience and were oriented toward the positive part of the narrative. I asked him to picture the first time he experienced the joyous sensation of his heart-pounding butterflies in his stomach: "If that feeling could be a color, what would it be? What would it smell like? Taste like? What texture would it be? What does it sound like?" He took those answers and created a digital collage to discharge some of those associations and give a visual language to the

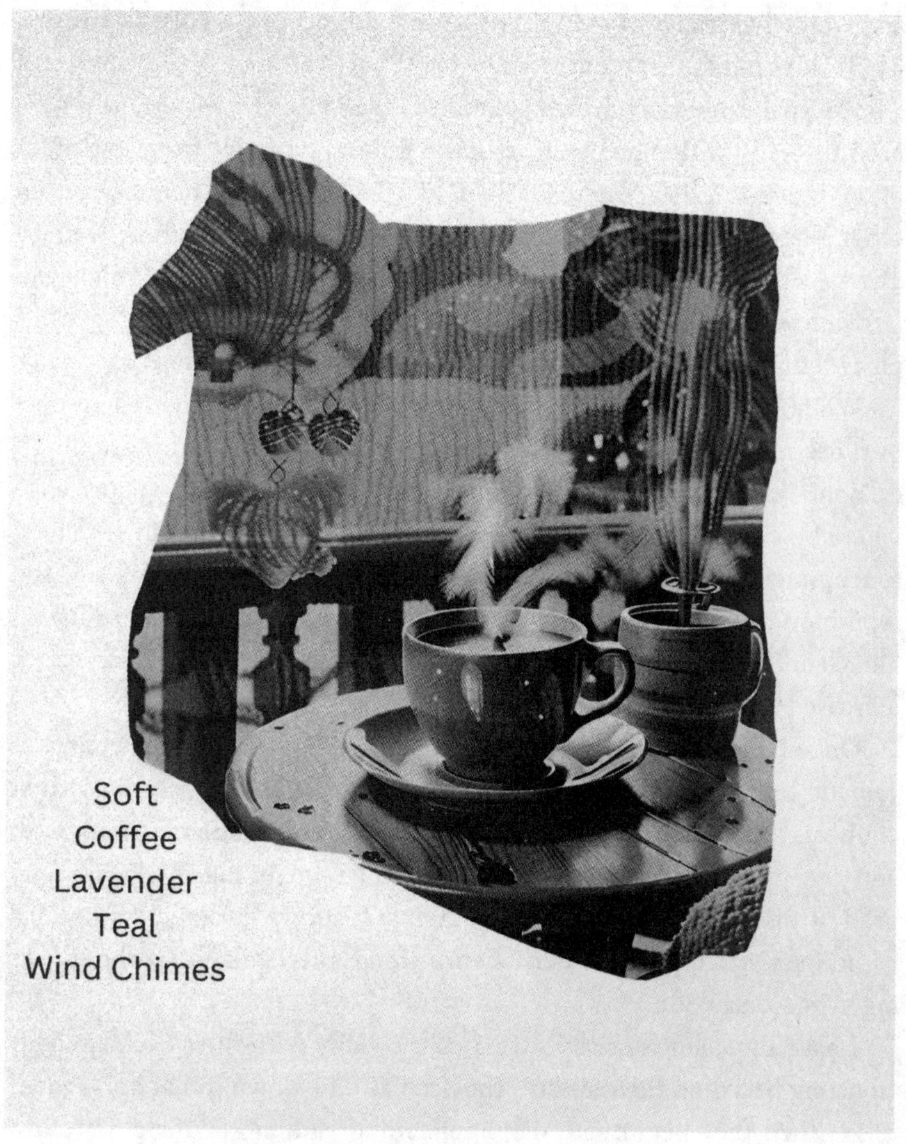

Figure 1. Sensory collage

experience. In creating the image, he wanted to weave in the colors lavender and teal, a representation of lavender as a smell, the taste of coffee or espresso, images that represented softness, and images that represented the subtle sound of wind chimes in the breeze. As he saw the personal and familial narrative come into physical existence, he could ask himself, where does our Queer identity come in? Where can I see the possibility of a brave space amid my body's reaction to past negative experiences? We used the sensory image he created as a grounding point from this point in the process. This is where I will often bring the client's narratives from other parts of the therapeutic work into our discussion about their piece of art. As the client looked at what he had made so far, I asked, "When you envision your Queer identity and what that means to you, where does this piece shift? Where do you experience new somatic symptoms?"

While discussing this narrative, the client started to experience some of those negative autonomic responses, so he stepped into more physical somatic reactions. I guided him through another sensory experience where he could look around the room and label what he could see, hear, touch, smell, taste, and what was present that could ground him. Using the repetition of the five, four, three, two, one grounding technique allowed him to find consistency, a sense of safety, and familiarity that allowed for increased regulation capacity.

Once he was grounded, he moved into a deep breathing exercise. In somatic breathwork, I suggest circular breathing along with music that connects to the narrative, bringing in the art's visual, the music's sound, and the breath's physical sensation. Circular breathing is a technique used by players of woodwind instruments. It allows for long, continuous breathing that supports sustainable breathing and regulation without risking hyperventilation.[15]

I have the client start by sitting comfortably with their back straight, adjusting based on their ability. They can also lie down if that helps them relax. Then they begin with diaphragmatic breathing, taking a few slow, deep breaths using their diaphragm. They inhale through their nose, allowing their abdomen to expand, and exhale slowly through the mouth. I then ask them to focus on the rise and fall of their belly, which helps anchor their awareness of their body. If the client cannot fully connect with their body, we may choose a spot on the wall, ceiling, or a bodily sensation that feels safe. Next I introduce elements of circular breathing. They fill their cheeks slightly with air during a steady exhale. As they approach the end of the exhale, they begin a slow, deliberate inhale through their nose while using the air stored in their cheeks to maintain a continuous, gentle flow. Over time, an increased focus can be on the seamless transition between exhale and inhale. Clients are encouraged to breathe slowly and steadily, aiming for a natural and unforced rhythm. The key is to avoid any strain. If they feel tension in their face or chest, they should ease back to normal diaphragmatic breathing and try again in a future session.[16]

Once this client felt that his nervous system was calmed, he moved into the identity piece of this work, which felt the most activating. This process took multiple sessions of practicing breathing techniques, examining the layered narratives, and reorienting to his initial sensory artwork. Creating repetition in the session and holding some space for predictability made it easier for this client to engage in the more profound work. As therapists, we need to both provide predictability and challenge the comfort zone. When the client was ready, we started to examine the romantic and sexual narratives that initially felt harder to discuss and express.

The client was moving into the pieces that were generally more difficult to verbalize, so I asked, "When you felt the feeling of romantic or sexual attraction, where did you feel it, and how did your body read that experience?" He shared that he could remember his heart beating fast and his chest tightening, and he struggled to differentiate the feeling from the first time he felt it during his initial trauma. He expressed that this association generally stopped him in his tracks: It felt challenging to move forward with pursuing relationships because he felt the need to run away rather than toward the person who brought up these feelings. When we dug deeper, he shared that while the need to run was there, he also felt butterflies in his stomach, his cheeks flushed, and his face would feel warm. When he tapped into those other sensations, he became aware that his nervous system and brain switched between *we need to be safe* and *this is new and exciting*. That subtle shift in his understanding of his somatic experiences helped him feel open to exploring these new narratives.

We began with the *new and exciting* feeling as he felt most called to that shift in his understanding of himself. So I asked, "What does it mean to know you are attracted to a Queer person and that they are Queer rather than assuming you would be with a cis-hetero woman?" He found this question complex. He reflected on how the trauma narrative was coming up for him. Growing up without acceptance from his family was part of the initial flight reaction. We paused and did some breathing and re-oriented to the reality that his personal trauma narrative and the sociopolitical narratives about Queer people would come up in this process. From this point, I asked if we could shift the focus to his discovery of his younger self and how that was the part that might be reacting. That resonated with him and our work, so we added music to the experience. We started by listening to songs that made him feel strong and empowered. I asked him to name a song that reminded him of this initial experience of attraction. What song would he hear in a coffee shop or driving in the car, and would he feel like he was back at that initial moment of attraction? After some thought, he labeled "Crazy Little Thing Called Love" by Queen. We listened to the song together once and then pulled out his sensory artwork (Figure 1). He examined it while listening to the song and expressed seeing a connection between the artwork and the music. I asked him to make some movements to the song and see what feelings came up for him and what shifted in his body.

Integrating music in the therapeutic process catalyzed the client's shift from fear to excitement. Music is an incredibly potent medium in trauma therapy, with its capacity to evoke memory and emotion. Sound provided by familiar or empowering songs can facilitate a reconnection with a part of the self that may have been silenced by trauma. Combining music with movement opens up further channels for expressing and reprocessing emotions.

Movement can include dance and mindful movement practices, which have been shown to foster a deep connection between body and mind. In the context of Queer bodies narratives, movement can serve as a reminder of the inherent dynamism and fluidity of identity. When clients can move freely to a piece of music that resonates with their experience, they are not only expressing emotions that may be difficult to verbalize. They are also physically enacting a narrative of liberation. Physically embodying change reinforces the idea that healing is both bodily and emotional. The multimodal integration of sensory art, music, and movement in therapy addresses the complexity of trauma on multiple levels. By engaging different senses simultaneously, the client can bridge the gap between the unconscious bodily memory and the conscious narrative. Reintegrating these experiences can lead to profound shifts in self-perception and identity reconstruction.

As he moved, he shared that there was a shift from wanting to run away from the feeling to running toward it, that at that moment, he could read the difference between his nervous system's responses to trauma and joy. This shift made it easier for him to label that the flight was not just about familial trauma, but the greater fear of how Queer narratives are oppressed politically on a scale that is both national and global, as well as fear of all the repressed memories and intense emotions that come up in trauma work. The fear was not just his familial trauma, rejection, or bodily disconnection; it was the reality that, in our work, there would be a continuous and ever-present trauma that we would both be sharing in a parallel process. This decisive moment in our work together changed us as people.

A continual struggle against silencing, erasure, and pathologization marks the historical context of Queer narratives. For much of modern history, Queer bodies were subject to both legal and social mechanisms designed to oppress and marginalize. These systems of control manifested in overt violence, institutional discrimination, and covert cultural messaging that devalued non-normative bodies and desires. Historians and cultural critics have documented how the suppression of Queer narratives not only robbed individuals of their self-expression but also obscured the rich and diverse heritage of Queer communities.

Over time, however, acts of resistance and reclaiming of identity have transformed these silenced voices into potent narratives of survival and resilience. Activism in the 1960s and 1970s, along with the emergence of Queer theory, has provided a language to articulate the pain and resistance experienced by Queer people.[17] This resurgence of narrative has fostered spaces where individual experiences of joy, trauma, and identity coexist. Therapists working with Queer clients often find that rearticulating these narratives in the safety of the therapeutic space becomes a revolutionary act, one that challenges historical norms and paves the way for healing.

I was struck by the profound importance of understanding our sociopolitical narrative in such moments. Each person lives within a system, or systems, built on inequities, disproportionate power dynamics, violence, and oppression. Denying that is denying ourselves the truth of our traumas and the truth of the collective traumas we hold. For example, much of documented Queer history was destroyed during World War II when Nazis burned down the Institut für Sexualwissenschaft, erasing Magnus Hirschfeld's works on Queer history, including the spectrum of gender.[18] That event speaks to the collective trauma that the Queer community continues to face, and speaks volumes to the history since WWII, culminating in the 2020s. Transphobia and homophobia are steadily on the rise and the Queer community is experiencing cumulative trauma. As a result, a shared set of trauma responses develops within Queer people across the US (and the world). Cumulative and shared cultural trauma are real experiences that affect people on a deep, fundamental level and need tending to. When these feelings arise, the response ranges from shutting down to feeling angry, scared, depressed, or uncertain. With shared trauma, the body can experience the same triggers as it does under any other trauma. The difference is that it is largely a collective experience based on shared identity. Shared trauma is a specific kind of parallel to individual narratives that can be both comforting and simultaneously soul-crushing.[19]

In this case example, the client was interested in exploring Queer history further to develop an understanding of the broader narrative that affected them. It is essential for us, as therapists, to recognize that trauma is not confined to the individual; it is transmitted across generations and embedded in cultural practices and historical narratives. Research in epigenetics suggests that the scars of trauma may be visible not only in memories and behaviors but also in the very structure of our DNA, passed down as a silent testament to historical suffering. For Queer clients, this means that their embodied experiences are interwoven with the stories of countless others who have fought against oppression. Acknowledging this intergenerational continuity can profoundly validate and empower clients to reclaim a narrative of resilience and hope.

Epigenetic research also suggests that trauma can lead to biological changes that are inheritable. The transmission of these biological markers means that the effects of trauma can persist long after the original event, influencing how subsequent generations experience stress and resilience. Such research underlines the importance of addressing both the psychological and the somatic dimensions of trauma in therapeutic work. By understanding that the body holds stories that may not be accessible to conscious memory, therapists can validate experiences that clients might otherwise struggle to articulate.[20]

With this client, this is where we discussed the reality of intergenerational trauma and how it could be something passed down within a family, such as his rejection trauma from his family, and could also be a collective trauma passed down through a group of people someone is a part of. "Intergenerational trauma" refers to the transmission of the effects of trauma from one generation to the next, often due to historical or collective events such as war, slavery, genocide, colonization, transphobia, homophobia, xenophobia, or systemic violence. The emotional, psychological, and physical impacts of trauma can be influence how future family members think, feel, and behave. Intergenerational trauma is transmitted through multiple domains, including psychological and emotional, behavioral, cultural and social, and biological.[21]

The emotional and psychological impacts of trauma, such as anxiety, depression, and post-traumatic stress, can be inherited through family dynamics, attachment styles, and coping mechanisms. For instance, a parent who experienced severe trauma may unknowingly pass on a heightened stress response, anxiety, or difficulty managing emotions to their children. Clients with trauma may develop coping strategies, such as avoidance or detachment, that they later model for their children. These behaviors may become ingrained as family norms and continue to influence how future generations deal with conflict, stress, and emotional regulation. In some cases, entire communities carry the weight of intergenerational trauma that stems from historical oppression or violence, which continues to shape their collective identity, cultural practices, and social structures. This is the kind of trauma, and trauma responses, we are seeing during the current time period.[22]

Research in epigenetics has shown that the biological effects of trauma can affect gene expression in ways that may be passed down. For example, trauma can alter how genes are expressed in response to stress, which might make offspring more susceptible to certain mental health conditions or stress-related diseases, even if they have not experienced trauma directly. The part of the brain that regulates the body's stress response, the hypothalamic-pituitary-adrenal axis, can be dysregulated by trauma, and that dysregulation can be passed down, making subsequent generations more vulnerable to anxiety, depression, or other stress-related conditions. All of this is caused by historical and systemic trauma, where groups and communities have experienced widespread violence or oppression and continue to carry its scars. Cultural loss results in disconnection from artistic practices, which can lead to a lack of cultural grounding for subsequent generations, further compounding the effects of trauma.[23] This client found this level of education on the topic helpful in conceptualizing how they could incorporate this kind of narrative into their work.

I often use a series of expressive art therapy techniques to address inherited trauma. One is called El Duende process painting, where people continuously paint on a canvas in layers, responding to bodily sensations and an inner knowing. Clients have an opportunity to confront their inner struggles and allow the creative process to transform their therapeutic experience. This process forces the client to divest from the aesthetics of traditional studio arts by focusing on emotions, physical sensations, and what symbols, colors, and experiences call to them in the creative process. It also taps into the cultural stories of "El Duende," who are Hispanic folklore creatures known for their passion, creativity, protective instincts, expression, and authenticity. These feelings and experiences are integrated into the artistic process.[24]

With this client, I used a canvas on the larger side so he could engage in the process and use their whole body to create. Tapping into the internal response to a national narrative enabled the client to expel the images, feelings, and nervous responses. The client wanted to start with a collage for this piece, so they began with some tissue paper and glue. As they glued it down, they talked about how fragile the paper felt, how easily it ripped, and how simple white tissue paper felt. He compared the tissue paper to skin, how fragile the human body is, and how it reminded him that we all have that fragility in common. It inspired him to want to add elements that reminded him of the human body. In the next session, he came in excited to dive into the process and brought pipe cleaners. He discussed being in an art supply store and seeing blue and red pipe cleaners, which reminded him of veins.

Diving into that association, he said in between our sessions, he had been thinking of the fragility of the human form and how so often he felt pushed, shoved, and manipulated to conform, including delaying his transition. This was a big moment in his Queer body narrative work. He began weaving the pipe cleaners together to make it look like a vein system and then glued them down. When he stopped, he turned to me and said, "You know this also reminds me of tree roots, something that has been in the ground long before us and will be long after." This was a powerful moment for us at work. He related the fragility and strength together, which felt like a beautiful metaphor for the Queer experience. Over the subsequent few sessions, he continued to collage red and white tissue paper over the pipe cleaner layer. His final collage layer was a series of white pieces of tissue paper. He then took markers and began writing five phrases over and over: *I am Queer enough. Trans lives matter, even if they do not say so. I am worthy. I am my ancestors. You will not erase us.* He found this part of his process incredibly emotional and would pause to practice breathing or move his body, organically integrating previous therapeutic experiences.

His sustained engagement with art therapy opened avenues for deep healing. Rituals had become an integral part of the therapeutic process.

Repeated acts of creative self-expression are pivotal; they transform what might initially be raw, unrefined emotion into a structured, empowered language that the body and mind can both understand and celebrate. From his simple grounding exercise to an elaborate multi-session art directive, rituals help create a structure within which clients can safely process trauma. The repetition inherent in rituals allows clients to reclaim a sense of order in a life that may feel chaotic or fragmented. Whether through the methodical layering of paint or the repeated practice of circular breathing, the ritualistic nature of these activities anchors the client in the present moment. It fosters an environment of safety and predictability. In many cultural traditions, rituals are closely connected to healing, symbolizing rebirth, transformation, and connection to something more significant than the individual. For Queer clients, whose narratives often involve experiences of isolation and alienation, engaging in a ritualistic process can be compelling.

Furthermore, integrating ritual into therapy underscores the idea that healing is not linear. Healing is cyclical and recursive, and often requires revisiting and reworking past experiences until a new narrative can emerge. Predictable rhythms soothe the nervous system and foster a renewed sense of stability and continuity in one's identity. The client's careful attention to bodily sensations during these rituals, such as noticing the rhythm of their breath or the tactile quality of art materials, helps ground them in the reality of their own embodied experience. Somatic awareness is key in countering dissociation and reclaiming the body as a site of strength and beauty.

Using the knowledge of rituals and their importance in the El Duende process allowed us to expand the process.[25] So in our next session, we reviewed the imagery and metaphors from the previous sessions and he looked through the art supplies to see what resonated for him. He began painting the next layer with black paint, covering the previous layers. In subsequent sessions, he began to make circular shapes using different pastel and neon colors. His body would often rock in a circular motion, getting lost in the creation flow (see Figure 2). During what became the second-to-last

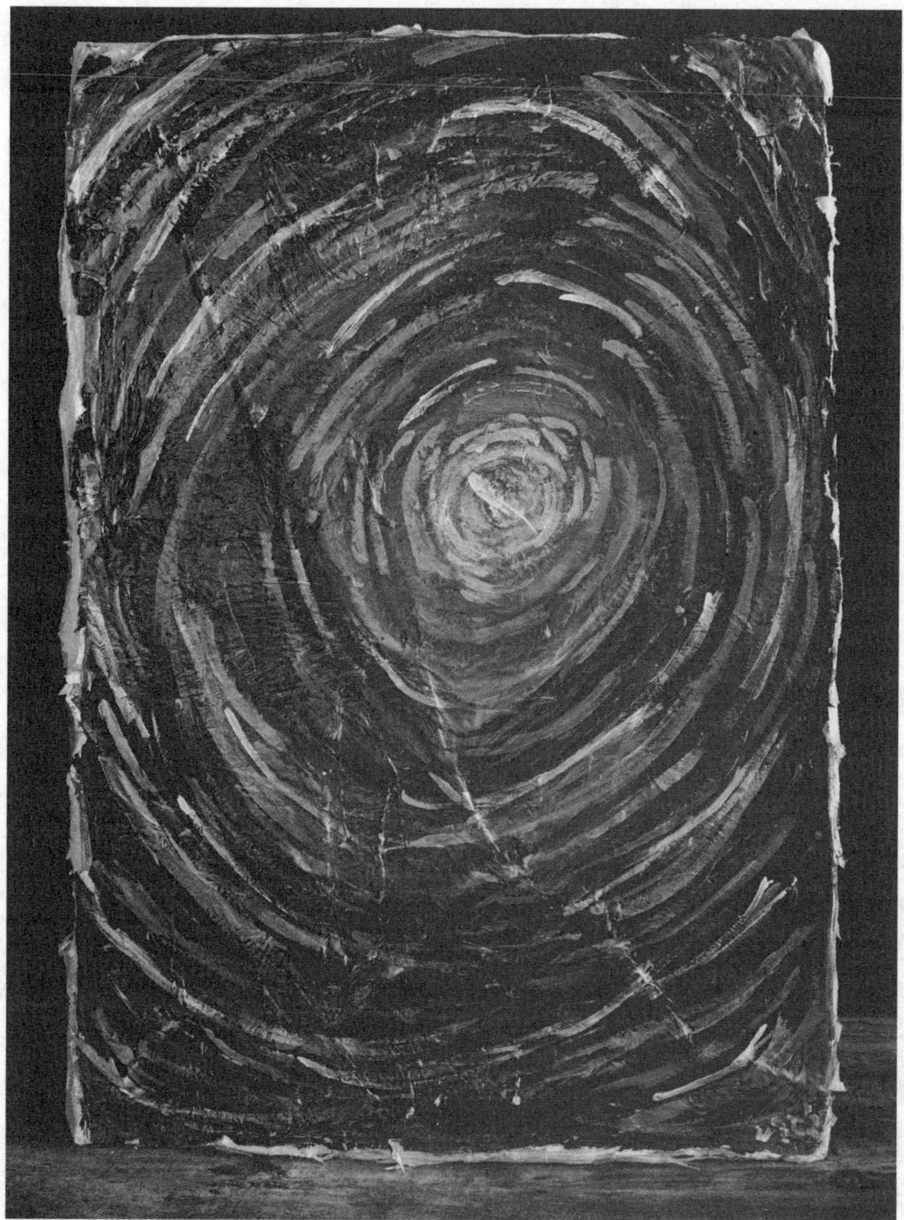

Figure 2. El Duende process painting

layer, he discussed wanting to incorporate herbs and dried flowers that he felt connected him to femininity. This became a rich discussion around what it meant to him to have part of his body's narrative encompass femininity when he had pressed so hard almost to erase femininity from his gender presentation. He shared that in this process, he no longer saw that part of himself as wrong or robbing him of being a man, but instead as an integrated part of himself that was equally part of his story. I showed him how to blend dried lavender, chamomile, rose petals, stone shards, and glitter into white paint, which he used around his circular shapes. He expressed the sensory experience of the smell of the dried herbs, which reminded him of our initial sensory work in sessions prior. In his final layer, he added dots that reminded him of stars and a feather he found outside.

When he was done, the client shared that when he looked at it, he felt small, like a speck in the narrative of the universe, and also felt expansive, like the colors simultaneously encompassed not just his narrative but all the Queer bodies and narratives that we may never hear or see but know are out there. He felt this process painting was ultimately a reflection of all his body narratives, his Queer narratives, and the realities that Queer bodies live under. These parallel narratives will not go away until our sociopolitical system changes in ways that would be revolutionary. Until then, as therapists, we can find ways to honor its existence, cope, and foster resilience for our Queer clients.

PRACTICE EXAMPLE

Process Painting and Collage as Affirmation

In a calm, private space, lay out a large canvas. Gather all materials: white and red tissue paper, glue, blue and red pipe cleaners, black, pastel, and neon paints, brushes or palette knives, dried lavender, chamomile, rose petals, stones or shards, glitter, a feather, and a fine-tip marker. Invite the client to begin with a sensory grounding, orienting to their surroundings through sight, sound, touch, smell, and internal taste, before settling into a few rounds of gentle circular breathing to steady the nervous system.

Together, articulate a personal affirmation or ancestral phrase to invoke the spirit of El Duende, raw authenticity, protective passion, and creative fervor. Then prompt the client to recall the early trauma of a pounding heart, noticing where that activation lives in their body, as they tear and collage white tissue across the lower canvas, speaking aloud about fragility and skin and naming any concurrent sensations.

As they shift attention to warm presence, they weave pipe cleaners into branching patterns over the tissue, exploring how vulnerability and lifeblood intertwine while breathing into the areas of safety they feel.

Then guide a seamless inhale–exhale into their conscious breath before they sweep black paint across the emerging imagery to symbolize hidden shame or a buried narrative, pausing after each stroke to observe any somatic shifts.

Uplifting music invites the client's body to sway as they paint large pastel and neon circles in rhythm with the beat, embodying joy and empowerment through whole-arm movement. Noticing the aroma of herbs, they mix dried lavender, chamomile, rose petals, stones, and a touch of glitter into white paint and apply this scented layer around the circles, attending to where calm or warmth arises in their chest or belly.

Finally, they repeatedly inscribe chosen affirmations across the surface and affix a single feather as a symbol of connection and expansiveness. To close, sit side by side with the client taking in the finished piece, inviting them to name the sensations they experience now, whether grounding, ease, or gentle activation, while reflecting, verbally or in writing, on where in the artwork they feel drawn toward rather than compelled to flee from, anchoring new insights about their Queer and ancestral narratives in both body and image.

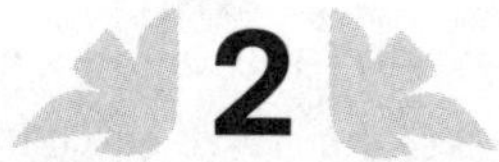

2 Body Liberation and Harm Reduction

Many of my clients, in their journey of existing in a Queer body, have faced inherent struggles. What does it mean to be in a Queer body? What does living in a body that holds multiple marginalized intersections mean? To be in a body that challenges the status quo of cis-hetero normativity? The answers are complex and cannot be stated in simple sentences or addressed in a single therapy session. The evolution of what it means to live in a Queer body cannot be disentangled from the historical, cultural, and social shifts that have led us to this moment. Today, the Queer body is more than just a site of identity, and it is a living testament to the ongoing evolution of self-expression. Throughout history, bodies deviating from normative expectations have been met with overt and subtle forms of discrimination. In the modern era, while acceptance and visibility have gradually increased, many people still face systemic challenges that reinforce the notion that there is a "right" way to be or exist. The struggles for many of my clients are intertwined with these broader societal narratives that seek to contain and regulate their existence. It is here that expressive art and somatic therapists play a crucial role. These therapists have the unique opportunity to adopt frameworks that support clients in expanding their Queer body narrative, and in doing so, they help clients develop a deeper understanding of themselves.

Living in a Queer body means inhabiting an identity that is layered with intersections of race, gender, ability, socioeconomic status, and more. Each of these dimensions brings its own set of challenges, triumphs, and unique forms of expression. For example, a Queer person of color may grapple with the dual pressures of combating racial stereotypes while also resisting heteronormative expectations. In many cases, the intersectionality of these identities means that the societal barriers are compounded, which creates a complex web of marginalization that is not easily addressed by one-dimensional approaches.

At the heart of an individual's unique experience lies the embodied experience, how the body is both a vessel of personal identity and a battleground for societal norms. The Queer body is often subject to scrutiny, regulation, and violence, yet it is also a site of profound creativity, resistance, and transformation. Existing outside society's prescribed norms is not merely political defiance but a deeply personal act of reclamation. In its natural state of diversity, the body becomes an expression of a self that refuses to be boxed into categories that were never meant to contain it. Herein lies the power of expressive art and somatic therapy.

Expressive art therapy offers a unique space for individuals to explore and articulate their inner worlds in a manner that transcends traditional verbal communication. Through painting, movement, music, and dance, clients can access parts of their identity that might be hidden beneath layers of social conditioning and internalized shame. The process of creating art can serve as both a mirror and a window, reflecting the complexities of a Queer identity while also offering a glimpse into alternative ways of being. In creation, clients are not just externalizing their pain or joy; they are reconstructing their narrative, allowing themselves to see their body as a site of possibilities rather than oppression.

Somatic therapy, on the other hand, directly engages with the body's physical experience. This modality recognizes that trauma, societal stress, and internal conflict are stored in the body as much as they are stored in the mind. Using techniques that focus on bodily sensations, movement, and the physical manifestation of emotion, somatic therapists help clients reconnect with a part of themselves that may have been disowned or fragmented. This approach is compelling for those who have experienced bodily erasure or objectification. It provides a pathway to reclaim bodily autonomy and establish embodied safety. In a society where the Queer body is frequently subjected to external control, be it through discriminatory practices, invasive medical procedures, or violent hate crimes, reclaiming ownership over one's physical self is not just an act of radical self-love but a political act of resistance.

Both expressive art and somatic therapies allow for a kind of narrative re-authoring, where clients are encouraged to see themselves as creators of their own story. This creative act of re-narration shifts the focus from what has been taken away or imposed upon the individual to what can be built from within: a resilient, vibrant, and profoundly authentic sense of self. The transformative power of narrative re-authoring is a key aspect of the healing process. Contemporary understandings of gender and sexuality emphasize the fluidity of both identity and the body, offering liberation through continual self-reinvention while also challenging rigid social categories. Living in a Queer body thus becomes an ongoing, transformative journey of internal discovery and external expression.

The complexity of this journey is often compounded by the external pressures to conform to a binary or normative ideal. The constant negotiation between one's internal sense of identity and the external demands of society can lead to feelings of isolation, anxiety, and even disconnection from one's body. Many of my clients describe a persistent tension, a sense of being caught between who they are and what society expects them to be. This tension is not quickly resolved; it requires a supportive and robust therapeutic framework that validates their experiences and honors their struggle. Here, the work of expressive art and somatic therapy is invaluable, as it creates a space where these tensions can be acknowledged, explored, and ultimately integrated into a more cohesive sense of self, reassuring those witnessing the client that the process is effective.

The very act of living authentically can be seen as a political statement, a refusal to submit to the oppressive dictates of cis-hetero normativity. This defiance, however, comes at a cost. Time and time again, Queer bodies are on the front lines of societal battles over rights, representation, and recognition. The struggles are not solely personal but deeply embedded in the fabric of social and political life. Advocacy, art, and therapy intersect in powerful ways to create personal healing and social change. When individuals reclaim their bodies through creative and somatic practices, they contribute to a more significant cultural shift that challenges the status quo and redefines what it means to be human.

For those who exist at the crossroads of multiple marginalized identities, the process of self-acceptance and bodily reclamation must also contend with the legacies of racism, sexism, ableism, and other forms of discrimination. These factors shape how one experiences one's body and the world. The confluence of various identities necessitates a therapeutic approach that is both holistic and nuanced, one that can address the layered realities of each client's life. In this context, the work of therapists who employ expressive art and somatic modalities is not only therapeutic but also an act of resistance against an oppressive system that seeks to divide and diminish.

Ultimately, the journey toward understanding and embracing a Queer body is a multifaceted and ongoing process of challenges, triumphs, setbacks, and breakthroughs. It requires the courage to face deep-seated fears and the resilience to forge a new path forward. For those who dare to live authentically, their body becomes a powerful medium of self-expression and social change. Thus, the work of embracing and expanding the Queer body narrative is not just about individual healing; it is about collective transformation. It calls all who have ever felt marginalized, erased, or misunderstood to reclaim their stories, celebrate their uniqueness, and contribute to a future where everybody is honored for their beauty and resilience. Through this work, the boundaries of what it means to be Queer continue to expand, inviting us all to imagine a world where diversity is not merely tolerated but celebrated as the very essence of what it means to be human.[1]

We can reframe our expanded understanding of what it means to live in a Queer body today by centering two critical frameworks: body liberation and harm reduction.

Body liberation is a revolutionary praxis that invites us to divest from the idea that individuals owe society a specific presentation or narrative about their body. It rejects the notion that bodies must adhere to singular, visual narratives and challenges the binary of "good" versus "bad" bodies. In parallel, harm reduction provides a framework that does not solely focus on abstinence from harmful practices or behaviors. Instead, it acknowledges the pervasive and systemic harm embedded in our social, political, and cultural institutions. Together, these approaches offer possibilities for reimagining body image work with Queer clients. They provide tools for therapeutic transformation that honor the complexity of embodied experiences.[2]

Rewriting the Body's Narrative

Body liberation recognizes the body as a dynamic canvas that reflects both the beauty and the pain of lived experience. It offers a lens through which to see the body as an ever-evolving text, full of layers that intersect with identity, memory, desire, and cultural context.[3]

Historically, non-normative bodies have been subjected to various forms of control, ranging from medicalization and surveillance to outright violence. For centuries, dominant power structures have marked Queer bodies as deviant or dangerous. The legacy of this control is evident in the persistent societal emphasis on conformity and the marginalization of bodies that do not fit neatly into prescribed categories.[4] But over time, resistance to these oppressive structures has also taken shape. Social movements and Queer activism have been playing crucial roles in reclaiming space and identity. The advent of Queer theory and intersectional feminism further complicated traditional understandings of identity by emphasizing that bodies are not merely physical vessels but are also sites of political struggle and cultural expression. As such, body liberation is deeply entwined with political resistance; it is both an individual and collective act of defiance against structures that seek to limit human potential.

One of the most transformative aspects of body liberation is its ability to rewrite the body's narrative. It opens up a multiplicity of narrative possibilities beyond oppression or marginalization. For Queer clients, this means that the story of their body is no longer linear or predetermined by external forces. Instead, they can understand their body's experiences as a rich tapestry of intersections, each representing different aspects of identity, trauma, joy, and resilience.[5]

In therapeutic settings, narrative re-authoring is incredibly potent. It helps clients move beyond internalized messages of inadequacy or shame, which are often the byproducts of societal oppression. Through techniques like storytelling, movement, and visual art, clients are encouraged to explore the full breadth of their bodily experiences. In doing so, they begin to see their body as a vibrant expression of their unique life journey.

Central to the practice of body liberation is challenging the dominant visual narrative that bodies are meant to be seen in one specific way. For decades, mainstream media, fashion, and cultural narratives have propagated images of what bodies should look like. These images often glorify a narrow standard of beauty and fitness, leaving little room for diversity or deviation. In contrast, a liberatory praxis compels us to recognize that beauty is multifaceted and that everybody tells a unique story.[6]

Queer clients frequently encounter pressure to conform to standards that not only misrepresent their experiences but also contribute to harmful body-image issues. By integrating body liberation into therapy, therapists can help clients deconstruct these unrealistic ideals and rebuild their self-image based on authenticity and self-acceptance. This process involves critical reflection on how media and culture shape our understanding of beauty and the implementation of practices that foster self-compassion and bodily pride.

The binary of "good" versus "bad" bodies is another restrictive narrative that body liberation seeks to dismantle. This dichotomy suggests that some bodies are inherently worthy while others are not, a notion that has historically marginalized those who deviate from dominant norms. In a liberatory framework, all bodies deserve respect and care, regardless of how they align with societal ideals.

Therapists working with Queer clients can leverage this understanding by creating safe spaces where clients can explore their body without judgment. Through expressive art or somatic practices, the goal is to help individuals cultivate a sense of intrinsic worth independent of external validation. This means challenging the internalized voices conditioned to judge and reject aspects of their physical self and replacing them with narratives of strength, resilience, and inherent dignity.

Establishing a liberatory environment involves several key practices. The first is the affirmation of identity. Therapists must be well-versed in the language and cultural nuances of Queer identities. This includes understanding the unique challenges and strengths that come with being Queer, as well as recognizing the diverse narratives that clients bring to therapy.

The second practice is inclusivity and intersectionality. A liberatory space respects the full spectrum of intersecting identities. Therapists should actively work to validate the experiences of clients who are also navigating racism, ableism, and other forms of marginalization.

The third is collaboration and client autonomy. Therapists should collaborate with clients to co-create the therapeutic process, rather than imposing a fixed framework, to ensure their work aligns with the client's needs, experiences, and goals.

Finally, there is safety and containment. A liberatory praxis must also address the real-world risks that many Queer clients face, including discrimination and violence. Creating a space that feels physically and emotionally safe for clients is essential for effective therapy; it also brings an aspect of harm reduction into this work.[7]

Harm Reduction for Queer Clients

Harm reduction is a framework that originated in the context of substance use treatment. However, its principles apply to a wide range of therapeutic contexts, including work with Queer clients on body-image issues. At its essence, harm reduction is about meeting clients where they are, acknowledging the realities of their lived experience, and supporting them in ways that minimize harm without demanding immediate or total change.[8]

For many Queer individuals, harm is not an isolated event but a continuous experience embedded in everyday interactions. The cumulative impact of microaggressions, overt discrimination, and systemic injustice leaves its mark on both the body and the psyche. Harm reduction recognizes this ongoing reality and works to mitigate its effects. It validates people's experiences of harm and seeks to empower clients by providing them with tools for managing and reducing further harm.[9]

In a therapeutic context, harm reduction involves several key strategies. Validation and empathy are the first aspects in any harm reduction approach; they acknowledge the very real harm that clients have experienced or may experience. For Queer clients, this means recognizing that their struggles with body image are not personal failings but the result of systemic inequities. Harm reduction also shifts the focus from a deficit-based change model to a client-directed one. Clients are empowered to set goals, develop alternative coping strategies, or explore their body through art and movement. From here, we utilize incremental change, recognizing that transformation is often a slow and nonlinear process. Harm reduction advocates for small, manageable changes. This gradual approach respects the pace at which clients feel safe to engage with painful experiences. This allows us to use alternative care models, because the traditional medical models may not align with the needs of Queer clients, particularly those who have experienced harm through medical or psychiatric institutions. Harm reduction encourages exploring models of care that may include community-based interventions, peer support, and integrative therapies like expressive art and somatic work. Finally, a harm reduction approach prioritizes clients' physical and emotional safety. By creating nonjudgmental and supportive environments, therapists can help clients feel secure enough to explore complex topics without fear of re-traumatization.[10]

While body liberation emphasizes reclaiming bodily narratives and rejecting oppressive beauty standards, harm reduction ensures that this journey is cared for. The two frameworks are complementary: Body liberation provides the vision for a world where all bodies are celebrated, as harm reduction offers pragmatic strategies for managing the very real risks and pains associated with getting there. For Queer clients, this dual approach is particularly vital. Body liberation challenges the normative ideals that have contributed to their body shame and internalized oppression. And harm reduction acknowledges that their road to freedom has many obstacles but their journey can be supported by care. By integrating these frameworks, therapists can help clients navigate the complexities of transforming their body image in ways that honor their resilience and vulnerability.

Being client-centered is harm reduction. The therapeutic stance prioritizes the client's autonomy, well-being, and unique experiential truth. When a therapist intentionally creates a space where the client is placed at the center, they are making an ethical commitment to honor the client's inherent capacity for self-knowledge and self-determination. In such a space, the client is empowered to set the pace of their healing journey, determine the topics they wish to explore, and contribute to the educational process by sharing insights about what strategies or interventions resonate best with them. This level of collaboration and respect cultivates a safer environment where clients feel secure enough to explore what is authentic to them, both in their body and in the myriad narratives that shape their identities. My role is facilitator and guide, a person who holds a nonjudgmental space in which the client's narrative is welcomed and validated in all its complexity.

When therapists embrace a client-centered harm reduction model, they essentially affirm that the healing process is not linear or uniform but is as unique as each individual. In working with Queer clients, therapists need to acknowledge that the narrative of the Queer body is interwoven with various layers of identity, including intersections of race, gender, ability, and cultural background. Such intersections can contribute to diverse and sometimes conflicting internal narratives about one's body and self-worth. By placing the client at the center, therapists allow space for all these narratives to coexist rather than forcing them into a single, uniform story. This approach validates a client's multiple truths and experiences and recognizes that the healing process is about integrating these different facets rather than erasing or sidelining them. Transformation emerges from an environment where the client feels ultimately seen and heard, where their multiple stories can surface and intertwine.[11]

Being client-led means committing to minimizing harm by practicing transparency as therapists, sharing our rationale for suggested therapeutic interventions while inviting feedback. This openness demystifies the therapy process and fosters collaboration and trust. By deliberately slowing down the process, allowing creativity and genuine self-exploration to blossom naturally rather than leading the client to a resolution, we achieve harm reduction. In this waiting, in this patient holding of space, clients often find the courage to explore deeply embedded wounds and integrate their experiences into a coherent narrative of resilience and growth.

Moreover, a client-centered approach extends beyond the therapeutic encounter; it affects how clients interact with the broader world. When a therapist models respect for the client's pace and perspective, they indirectly equip the client with tools to advocate for themselves in other contexts. Clients learn to recognize their values and to resist external pressures that may otherwise push them toward harmful behaviors or self-neglect. Therefore, the therapeutic relationship becomes a microcosm of a more humane and just society, where each person's narrative is honored, and the potential for harm is continually minimized through empathy, understanding, and shared responsibility.

Being client-centered is an acknowledgment that every individual is the expert on their own body and experience, and that healing is best achieved when clients are allowed to lead the way. By creating a transparent and collaborative space, and adopting a slow, respectful approach to the therapeutic process, clinicians enable the richness of the Queer body narrative to coexist with other narratives. As Kuhfuß highlights, this approach honors the multiple truths and stories that each client holds, ensuring that harm is minimized and that the path to healing is as authentic and empowering as possible.

Case Example: Body Liberation and Harm Reduction with a Queer Client

One client who went through this work with me was a transgender, pansexual woman (she/her) in her late twenties who was Latina from a middle-class immigrant family. She came to me searching for support in navigating her family of origin, her connection to her body, and dysregulation in her mood. She fought hard for her family to accept her and shared that her teenage years were harrowing. At school she was made fun of for being Latina and for being the "weird boy who liked girl things." She discussed her struggles with gender dysphoria and how she would have to hide her experimentation with her hair and makeup so that her family would not find out. As she got older, her parents saw how she would get profoundly depressed and anxious in public, avoid social gatherings, and avoid anywhere she had to be seen by people because being perceived as "him" was too painful. Over time, her family was able to accept her and support her in participating in therapy. She began hormone replacement therapy (HRT).

By the time she started seeing me, she had socially transitioned and was still on HRT. Despite feeling she presented as a woman in public, she continued to experience intense dysregulation due to the sociopolitical climate surrounding gender and sexuality, as well as fears related to immigration, raids by federal Immigration and Customs Enforcement (ICE), and anti-Latina rhetoric under the current political climate. Her fears were very real and based on the sad reality that her body was somehow seen as threatening to others just by existing. This was coupled with the pain of being in a body that was assigned male at birth and her uphill battle to be accepted by her family, community, friends, and those around her. She lived with the knowledge that although she was born in the United States, she was a first-generation Latina and that very little could protect her from the things she feared the most. As a result, many therapeutic modalities were challenging for her because they involved a fully cognitive model: Change your thoughts to change your dysregulation. Those modalities failed her because her thoughts were not developmental insecurities; they were factual realities. She still struggled with somatic therapies because they were too body-based for her dysphoria. Rather than pushing the agenda that a specific regulation means stability, I asked the client how she felt about what a therapist would view as dysregulation and what she felt would be most supportive, knowing we cannot make the political climate or structure of oppression disappear.[12]

We discussed using harm reduction to alter the "therapeutic protocols," so they would fit what she needed rather than what the modality called for. She responded well to the idea that harm reduction could inform our initial approach and that she would be my guide for what is best for her, rather than me being seen as the expert, a "power with" versus "power over" approach. From here, I offered her suggestions about what I could provide, with the transparency that each of us offered different healing opportunities based on our individualized skill sets and comfort. Often, this is where the client and I have an open discussion. While I believe somatic and expressive art therapies are for everyone, that does not mean we need to use it or that this was the best fit for her. We agreed to try small things over sessions so she could decide what was best for her.

These therapies do help heal trauma, but if the client's body is not ready or does not feel safe enough, we can work together to use some of those modalities at their consent in a titrated way, which means gradually and carefully adjusting the intensity of the therapy to match the client's comfort level. With this client, I offered multiple curated options for directives, materials, somatic exercises, and more traditional treatments, so she could make an informed choice for her healing. She was open to trying a small body scan, so I gave her a paper with a basic body outline, which was not gendered, and colored pencils. I asked her to show me visually what she felt in her body when she felt oppressed. And I asked her to tell me what it felt like when she believed liberation and harm reduction were not possible for her. During this practice, she said that she had never felt heard until we began working together, and that previously she had felt forced into specific kinds of therapy that did not work for her and her body. It was through a client-centered approach that she was already able to re-envision what liberation could mean for her body and other Queer bodies like hers.

Throughout the body scan, I was quiet, letting her process the experience and see how she felt in her body. She chose colors, shapes, and patterns that best described her and her situation. In her art, she put colors and symbols in her legs, which she explained represented the constant need to run away or toward something rather than staying stagnant and thinking too hard. She covered her throat because she felt she had no voice outside therapy, or that her voice would be deemed somehow dangerous. Her genital area was covered partially by the gender dysphoria she experienced, and the reality that no matter how much she presented as a woman, she still lived in a world that devalued transgender women and people of color. Her body scan to observe what was dysregulating took two or three sessions. (See Figure 3.)

Here is where body liberation began to play out in this client's therapy. Through the body scan, we could move into what it means to be liberated from the societal narratives around bodies like hers. We began with the expressed feeling of running as if running from something. I asked her, "How would you feel if we reframed the need to run as a strength? A need to be autonomous, to save yourself rather than waiting to be saved?" This resonated with her as we looked at the body scan. We discussed how body liberation can be as simple as your legs or mobility aid carrying you somewhere you want to be.

Building on that moment, we delved deeper into the metaphor of movement as empowerment. In many traditional narratives, running is associated with fleeing, being chased, or with a sense of desperation. Yet when we reframe this action through the lens of body liberation, running transforms into a celebration of the body's capability, a declaration of independence.[13] In our session, I encouraged her to consider that every step her legs take is an act of self-determination. Instead of interpreting her physical movement as an escape from pain or danger, we began to see it as an assertion of agency. This subtle shift in perspective opened up a broader dialogue about how the body can be both a site of historical trauma and a tool for reclaiming autonomy.[14]

We explored the idea that societal narratives often dictate how our bodies should move and feel and what they are capable of. For many people, these narratives are suffused with expectations and limitations, ideas suggesting a "normal" way to experience bodily movement, a "right" way to exist. Body liberation invites us to challenge these norms by reimagining our physical selves as diverse and resilient. In our conversation, I shared that liberation is not about denying the pain or challenges her body has encountered but about recognizing its inherent value and potential. Her legs, for instance, are more than tools for escape; they are powerful instruments of transformation.

During the body scan, as we moved our awareness from the sensations in her legs to the broader map of her body, she began to identify areas where societal expectations had left their mark. We discussed how overt and subtle messages about what her body "should" be had created pressure to conform. I asked her to imagine a scenario where each part of her body was celebrated for its unique contribution rather than scrutinized for its

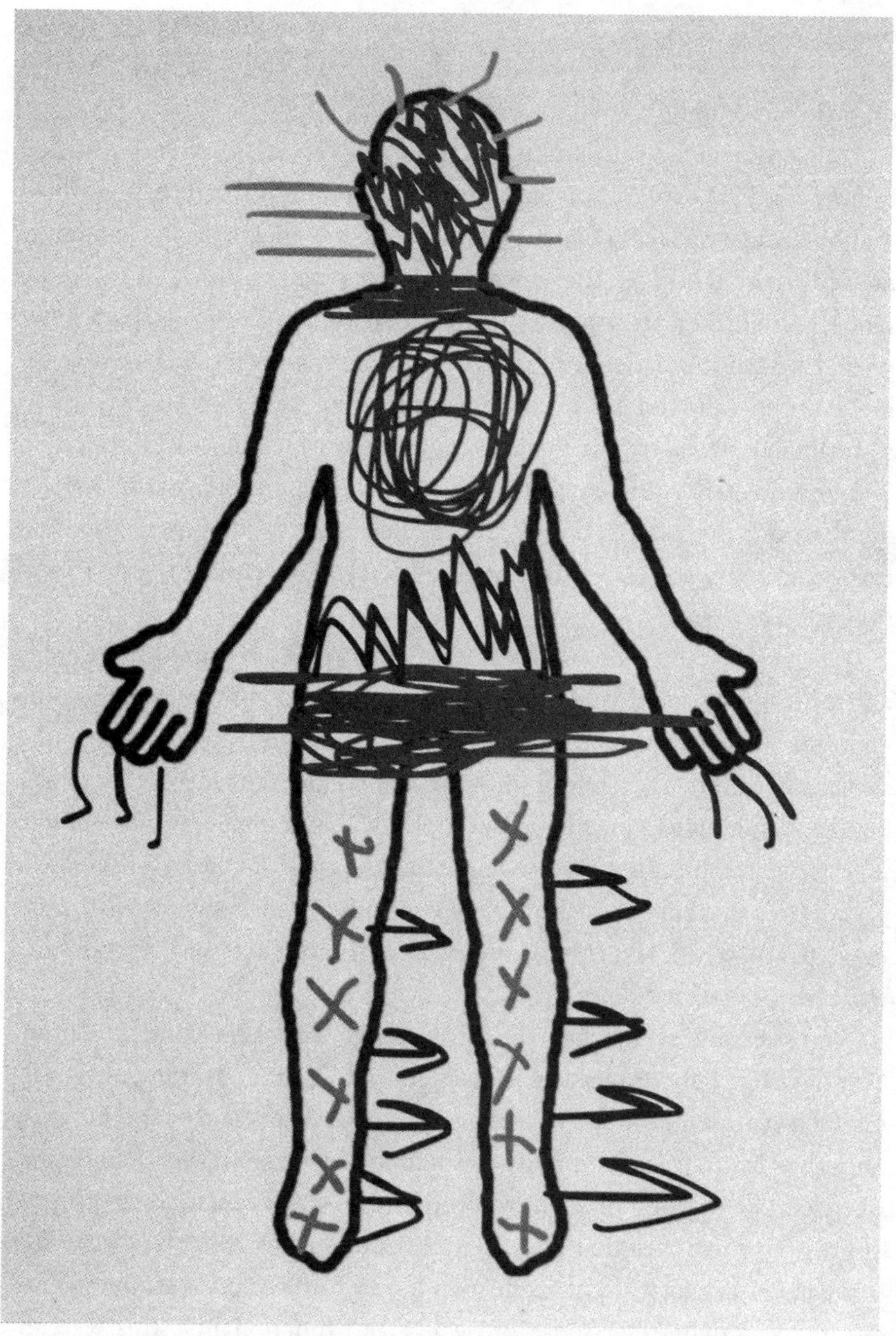

Figure 3. Body scan exhibiting feeling oppressed

perceived shortcomings. For example, if her legs could carry her to any desired destination, they represented the mechanics of movement and the promise of possibility.

As we deepened our exploration, the conversation naturally turned to how her past experiences had shaped her bodily narrative. In a world that has rigid standards of beauty, functionality, and worth, she had internalized many messages that devalue her very being. Through the body scan, we identified areas of tension and discomfort, as well as spaces that pulsed with potential energy reservoirs of strength that had been overlooked. I encouraged her to recognize those subtle signals and see them as resilience markers. For instance, a slight warmth in her calves could be reinterpreted as the energy of movement, a spark of life that propels her forward. In this way, body scanning became a tool for awareness and empowerment, mapping where pain resided and potential for growth and liberation existed.[15]

We also examined how the concept of running, reframed as a choice and a strength, could serve as a metaphor for everyday life. She could embrace the idea that every action she took was deliberate self-care and self-preservation. This shift in thinking helped her view her body not as a battleground but as a partner in her journey. In our dialogue, we explored practical ways she could honor this partnership. We discussed mindfulness practices that would allow her to tune in to her body's signals with compassion, and we looked at movement not as a chore but as a celebration of what her body could do.[16]

The session also touched on autonomy in a broader context. Autonomy is not just about physical movement but about reclaiming one's narrative in every aspect of life. Clients begin to assert control over their story once they learn to see their body as a source of strength rather than shame. I invited her to think of each movement as a small rebellion against the oppressive narratives that have long dictated her worth. Every time her legs carried her forward, it reaffirmed her right to be present, pursue her destiny, and define her sense of beauty and functionality. This was not merely a therapeutic intervention but a declaration of self-sovereignty.

In our continued work, we integrated expressive art into our sessions. I asked her to create a visual representation of liberation for her body: a collage, a drawing, or even a series of marks that captured the dual sensations of pain and possibility. The act of creation gave her a tangible medium to explore and express the internal transformations. As she painted or sketched, she narrated the story of her body: the scars of past expectations, the joy of newfound autonomy, and the ongoing journey toward self-acceptance. The boundaries between therapy and art dissolved in this creative process, allowing her to see her body as a canvas of history and hope.

The process of re-authoring her bodily narrative was deeply relational. It required us, as therapist and client, to engage in a dialogue that was both introspective and expansive. I emphasized that liberation is an ongoing, continuous dialogue with oneself. It has no definitive endpoint, only a series of evolving insights and practices. By holding space for her narrative without judgment, I demonstrated that harm reduction is not about leading a client to a particular outcome but facilitating a journey of self-discovery where they can explore their truths at their own pace.[17]

We also discussed how societal pressures can lead to a compartmentalization of the self, a disintegration of the body into parts that are judged, measured, and usually found lacking. Through our work, she began to see that her body could be reassembled into a narrative of wholeness, where each part, whether it felt strong or vulnerable, was integral to her identity. This holistic view is central to body liberation. It affirms that every sensation, every movement, and every scar is a testament to a life lived authentically. Liberation is not about erasing the past or ignoring pain; it is about integrating all of oneself into a coherent, self-affirming story.[18]

One of the most powerful moments came when she shared that the act of running, reinterpreted as a choice to be autonomous, had sparked a new understanding of self-reliance. Instead of feeling burdened by a need to escape, she began to see running as a dance with possibility, a way to navigate life on her terms. Her body scan revealed areas that once felt heavy with expectation were now lightened by the awareness that she was in control. This recognition was transformative: It validated her experiences and provided her with a renewed sense of empowerment.

Ultimately, exploring body liberation through the body scan became a metaphor for the larger work of healing. It was a reminder that liberation is both an internal and external process, a shift in perception that transforms the body from a site of conflict into a reservoir of strength and potential. It is about understanding that the narratives imposed by society are stories that we can rewrite. By reframing the need to run as a strength, we helped her see that autonomy and self-care are revolutionary acts in a world that seeks to diminish the value of the Queer body.[19]

Homing in on the concepts of body liberation and harm reduction, the client and I decided to engage in some art-making to discuss the integration of body liberation into their schema of being. She chose to paint, and walked around my studio looking at available materials. Her movements were deliberate, scanning the array of paints, brushes, and canvases with curiosity and contemplation. After a few moments of quiet consideration, she selected a vast canvas, around forty-eight inches tall, a decision that seemed significant in and of itself. When I asked about her choice, she mentioned wanting to work "bigger than herself," a symbolic way to move beyond the perceived limitations of her body and its relationship with space.

She chose dark colors, blacks, blues, and purples, deep and rich hues that seemed to resonate with something internal. As she began painting, she instinctively used large, curved brush strokes, sweeping the canvas with intention. Her movements were full-bodied; she reached up high, stretched her arms wide, and engaged her entire frame in the act of creation. Each stroke appeared almost like a dance, her body swaying with the rhythm of the brush. There was a rawness to her engagement, an immediacy that brought her fully into the present moment.

Sometimes she paused, stepped back, and examined the canvas, tilting her head as if deciphering a hidden message within her work. She occasionally moved away from the painting altogether, stretching her arms, rolling her shoulders, and taking deep breaths. The act of painting, which initially began as an exploration of body liberation, was already unfolding into a somatic practice.

At one point I asked her, "How does it feel to use your whole body to paint rather than feeling disconnected from it?"

She stopped, brush in hand, and thought for a moment. Then, contemplatively, she responded, "It feels . . . different. For once, my body isn't something I have to think about in terms of gender or dysregulation. It's just . . . part of making something."

Her voice carried a note of surprise, as if she were uncovering an unexpected realization.

This moment was profound. She stood still momentarily, letting her words' weight settle in. Then, as if propelled by this newfound understanding, she returned to her painting with renewed energy. She continued to paint the curved line, layering the purples and blues repeatedly, deepening the movement within the piece. Her process had a rhythmic quality, a repetition that seemed almost meditative. Over time, she introduced new colors, yellow, white, and gray, blending them into curved forms, allowing the colors to coexist dynamically.

As she worked, I noticed her breath had deepened, making her posture more fluid. Her actions evoked a sense of embodiment, as though she were allowing herself to fully inhabit her body in a safe, exploratory, and celebratory way.

I gently inquired, "What's happening for you as you add these new colors?"

She paused again, stepping back to observe.

"The darkness isn't bad," she murmured, almost to herself. "It's just the foundation. But I don't want it to be only that. I think . . . I need light, too."

She mixed a pale yellow with white and dipped her brush into the new hue, adding highlights to the curved lines. The contrast was striking, subtle, and impactful. The interplay between dark and light, movement and stillness, seemed to tell a story of integration, letting contradictions exist without negating one another.

This creation became a metaphor for body liberation, acknowledging struggle and resilience, allowing space for complexity rather than forcing a binary resolution. The process itself held meaning beyond the final image, illustrating the essence of harm reduction: meeting oneself where they are, without shame or pressure to conform to external expectations.[20]

As she continued, she spoke about memories of being told that her body was wrong, too much, too little, not fitting into the molds imposed by societal norms.

"I think that's why I used to make myself smaller," she admitted. "Like, physically trying to shrink, maybe if I took up less space, I'd feel better. But that never worked."

Her voice was steady, but with an undercurrent of emotion.

I nodded, giving space for the thought to exist.

"And now, you're choosing to take up space in this painting. In this room. In this moment."

She smiled faintly, then dipped her brush into a vibrant purple and added another sweeping curve, reinforcing the sense of expansion, and said, "Yeah. I think I am."

For the remainder of the session, she painted with quiet intensity and was fully engaged in creating. Her movements became even more fluid, and she sometimes stepped back to use her hands instead of the brush, smearing the paint with her fingers and feeling its texture directly against her skin. This tactile engagement deepened the connection, emphasizing the sensory experience of embodiment rather than just the visual outcome.

By the time she finished, the painting was a striking composition of movement, color, and emotion. The curved lines formed a layered, organic structure, like a tree's rings or the vast ocean's undulating waves. It was both grounding and expansive, representing transformation in real time.

She set down her brush, looking at the finished piece with quiet satisfaction.

"It's not what I thought it would be," she admitted. "But I think it's what I needed."

I nodded, acknowledging the significance of her words. "That's the beauty of this process. It doesn't have to be what you expected; it must be true to you."

She took a deep breath, stepping back one final time.

"I think I want to keep working on this. Not just the painting. The whole thing. Learning to take up space," she said. "Letting my body be mine."

With that, she gathered her things and left the painting to dry. It is a testament to her journey toward body liberation, one brushstroke at a time. (See Figure 4.)

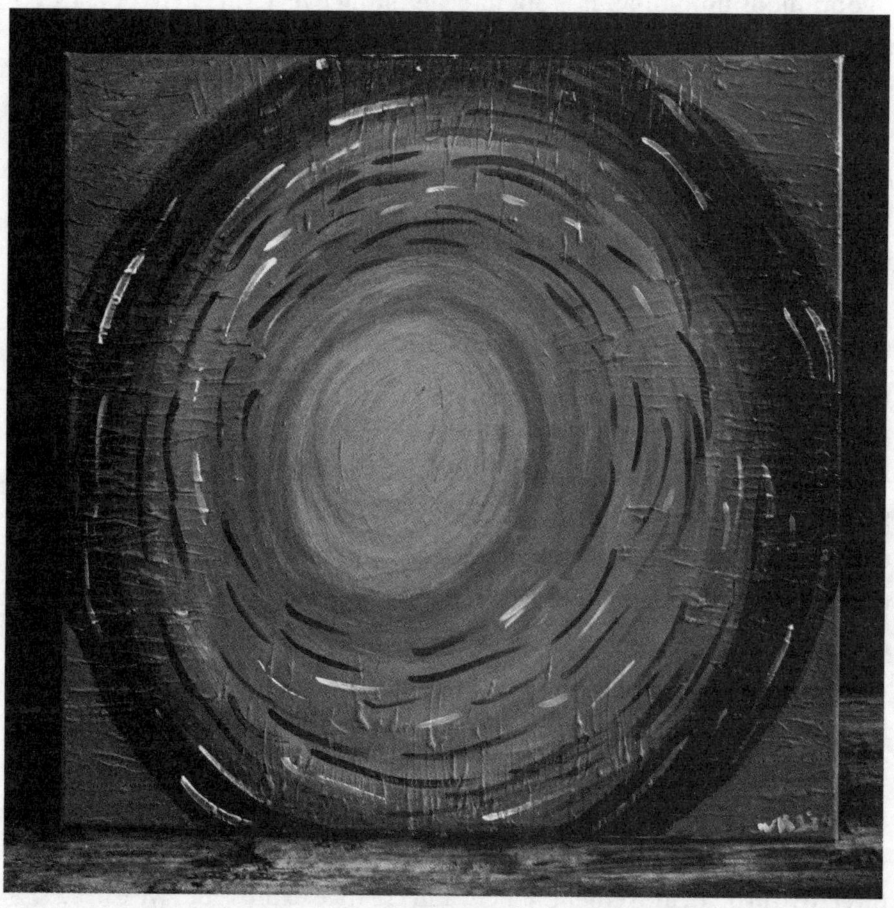

Figure 4. Body liberation painting

Combining body scanning, expressive dialogue, and creative exploration, this integrated approach illustrates how therapeutic practices can pave the way for profound transformation. When we honor the body's signals and reframe old narratives, we can create spaces of genuine liberation. In these spaces, the client is more than a recipient of therapeutic interventions; they are a co-creator of their healing journey. Their body, with all its scars and strengths, becomes a living narrative of resilience that defies oppressive societal expectations and embraces the fullness of self-determination.

In this process, we learned that body liberation is not a destination but a continuous unfolding. It is about celebrating every small victory, a step taken with intention, a movement that defies old narratives, and the courage to reimagine one's story. For her, and many others like her, the journey toward body liberation is a powerful affirmation of the right to exist fully and authentically, a daily act of reclaiming what has long been denied. It stands as a profound counterpoint to narratives that seek to limit the beauty and complexity of the Queer body.[21]

Embracing complex narratives is a powerful invitation to explore alternative ways of expressing our inner experiences and external realities. When we consider narratives not only as stories told in words but as embodied experiences, emotions, and memories, we open up a space for healing and growth that goes beyond the limitations of language. In doing so, we acknowledge that our experiences are not merely intellectual or verbal but also profoundly physical, emotional, and visual. This acknowledgment paves the way for using somatic and expressive art therapy as modalities that allow us to witness our stories through both the body and creative expression.[22]

Our body holds memories and emotions that words alone cannot capture. Traumatic events, for instance, can leave an imprint on the body that resists verbal articulation. Somatic practices in art therapy encourage us to reconnect with these stored memories by engaging with the body directly. Through movement, touch, and creative expression, we can access and process locked-away emotions. This embodied witnessing offers a path to healing because it releases tension, pain, and unresolved feelings nonverbally.[23]

When narratives are integrated into somatic practices, the body becomes an archive of lived experiences. A gentle movement sequence or a spontaneous gesture can communicate what might be too overwhelming to articulate verbally. As individuals engage in these practices, they witness their own embodied history, observing how specific postures, gestures, or sensations reflect personal narratives. In this way, the body is an active participant in creating and expressing its own story.[24]

Visual witnessing in expressive art therapy involves translating internal experiences into tangible forms, whether through drawing, painting, sculpture, or other artistic practices. This process externalizes internal narratives, thereby making the invisible visible. The creation of art becomes a mirror that reflects the complexity of one's inner life, including emotions, conflicts, and aspirations. Through art, feelings that are too deep or painful to articulate with words find a form of expression that is both containing and transformative.[25]

When narratives are embraced in this context, creating art becomes a dialogue between the self and the canvas, between internal experiences and external forms. Colors, shapes, and textures can nonverbally represent moods, memories, and sensations, inviting both the creator and the observer into a space of empathy and understanding. The artwork serves as a testament to the lived experience, a visual record that honors the complexity of human life.[26]

Therapists using somatic and expressive art therapy don't need to impose interpretations or guide the creative process too rigidly. Rather, they provide a supportive environment where clients feel safe exploring and expressing their narratives in diverse ways. This facilitative role involves acknowledging the uniqueness of each individual's story, helping them find modalities that resonate with their journey, and providing gentle prompts for reflection and discussion. Our role as therapists is to help the client integrate these experiences into a coherent narrative that fosters self-understanding and empowerment, while respecting the client's autonomy and pace.[27]

By taking a holistic view toward healing that includes one's cognitive, emotional, and physical layers, therapists and clients can explore how emotions manifest in the body and visual forms. Therapists might encourage clients to experiment with different forms of expression and to be open to the messages that arise from their body and creative practices. For instance, a client could start with a guided movement exercise that eventually transitions into a drawing session.[28] Or a client might notice that feelings of anxiety produce tightness in their chest, which can be gently released through mindful movement. At the same time, these feelings can be depicted in abstract art, such as with sharp lines and dark hues that eventually give way to lighter, more fluid forms as healing progresses. The dynamic interplay between bodily sensations and creative expression creates an interwoven narrative of healing, where every brushstroke or movement is an act of self-expression and a step toward recovery.

One of the most profound aspects of integrating narratives through somatic and expressive art therapy is the empowerment it brings to clients. When individuals are encouraged to explore their inner life through diverse modalities, they gain control over how their stories are told. This empowerment is particularly significant for those who have experienced trauma or marginalization, where narratives were imposed by external forces rather than emerging from within.[29]

In a therapeutic setting, empowered clients learn to trust their inner wisdom. They begin to see themselves not as passive recipients of their experiences but as active narrators who can shape their destinies. Creating art or engaging in mindful movement asserts this agency. It declares that their stories matter and that they have the power to rewrite the narratives that define them. Their shift in perspective fosters resilience, nurtures self-esteem, and opens up new pathways for personal growth. While individual healing is paramount, sharing these embodied and visual narratives is also immensely valuable. Group therapy sessions incorporating somatic and expressive art modalities allow individuals to witness each other's stories, creating a sense of solidarity and mutual support. In these shared spaces, personal narratives intersect with communal narratives that reflect diverse experiences and perspectives.

Collective witnessing can break down people's feelings of isolation. When participants share their artwork or movement experiences, they often discover common threads in their stories, struggles, joys, and transformative moments that resonate across individual differences. The shared experience of witnessing another's creative expression can validate one's own feelings and foster a deeper connection with others. This communal dimension enhances individual healing and contributes to broader social change by promoting empathy, understanding, and collective resilience. The benefits of embracing these narratives extend beyond the therapy room.

Once people see their stories as living, dynamic expressions of their inner selves, they can integrate these insights into their everyday lives. The skills learned through somatic and expressive art therapy, such as mindfulness, creative problem-solving, and emotional regulation, become tools for navigating the complexities of daily existence. For instance, mindfulness can help manage stress, creative problem-solving can enhance decision-making, and emotional regulation can improve interpersonal relationships.[30]

A person might do a simple sketch or a short movement routine during stressful moments to reconnect with themself. The practice reminds them that they have the capacity for creativity and healing. Over time, these modalities can transform how they interact with the world, fostering a more mindful, embodied, and authentic way of being. By embracing our narratives, we open the door to a multifaceted approach to healing that transcends the limitations of verbal expression. Through somatic and expressive art therapy, people can engage with their stories in ways that honor the full spectrum of human experience, body, mind, and spirit. These modalities facilitate personal healing and empower individuals to reclaim their agency, connect with others, and integrate their experiences into a richer, more authentic sense of self. Somatic and visual witnessing becomes a personal and collective act of resilience, paving the way for transformative healing and creative expression in everyday life.

PRACTICE EXAMPLE

Embodied Flow for Stress, Creativity, and Connection

Begin with a grounding phase in which the client finds a quiet, comfortable space, softens their gaze, and brings attention inward through a slow, mindful body scan from their feet upward, releasing tension with each exhale; they then anchor their nervous system by reaching their arms overhead on an inhale and, as they exhale, tucking their chin and gently rolling their spine down before articulating back up one vertebra at a time, noticing how each cycle deepens their sense of calm.

This naturally flows into an improvisational movement phase, where the client first sways in neutral to invite ease, then explores contrasting movement qualities, heavy versus light, direct versus indirect, sudden versus sustained, bound versus free, allowing each to inform how they might approach a real-life decision or creative challenge; as the client embodies these qualities, the therapist can pose questions like *What if I met this dilemma more lightly or more directly?* and welcome whatever solutions or metaphors emerge, integrating them afterward in words or sketches.

Finally, the client cultivates emotional regulation and relational attunement by placing a hand on their heart and another on their belly as they breathe in and out in resonance, extending their arms forward on each exhale as if offering warmth, and drawing them back on each inhale. All the while, the client can affirm silently, *I am open to understanding and to being understood*, so that heart-focused coherence can modulate their emotional arousal and enhance their capacity for empathy and connection. This seamless progression from interoceptive awareness to sensorimotor exploration to heart-centered breath offers a holistic, embodied approach to managing stress, unlocking creative insight, and deepening interpersonal harmony.

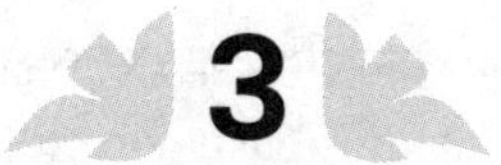

3 Combining Somatic and Expressive Art Therapies

Expressive art therapy harnesses the power of multiple expressive arts to address a wide range of therapeutic issues. Whether trauma, depression, an eating disorder, or struggles with identity, the use of the expressive arts combined with somatic therapy provides a unique path to healing by awakening deep-seated emotional and physical processes.[1] At its core, this modality asserts that creativity is not just an artistic pursuit but a vital language of the self that can transcend words and access parts of the mind and body that traditional talk therapies may not reach. Somatic and expressive art therapy is based on psychological theory, practice, and neuroscience underpinnings, which will help us understand the mind-body connection and how it is supported by this therapy. Most importantly, clients are able to document their lived experience, emotions, culture, spirituality, and existence.

Psychoanalytic Roots and the Unconscious

Building on Freudian and Jungian legacies, expressive art therapy leverages the symbolic potency of images and metaphors to bring unconscious content into awareness. Whereas Freud emphasized dream analysis and free association, the art therapist facilitates a "free creation" process: Clients are encouraged to engage with materials without censoring impulses, allowing latent themes, such as unresolved conflicts or archetypal patterns, to surface. Jung's notion of the collective unconscious further undergirds this work; when clients draw common symbols, they tap into shared human motifs that can catalyze deep psychological resonance.

Humanistic psychology's emphasis on self-actualization and innate growth potential finds clear expression as part of the expressive therapies continuum (see Figure 5). Carl Rogers's person-centered approach, marked by unconditional positive regard, empathy, and congruence, translates into the therapist's stance in expressive modalities: The studio becomes a nonjudgmental field where clients experiment with forms and colors as they would with aspects of the self. Existential themes, freedom, responsibility, and meaning-making often emerge organically as clients craft narratives through art, grappling with questions of identity, purpose, and autonomy.

Transpersonal psychology extends the therapeutic horizon beyond the individual's ego, embracing spiritual or trans-spiritual experiences. In expressive art therapy, this may manifest as visionary imagery, encounters with "inner guides," or a sense of connection with something greater than oneself. Techniques such as guided imagery, painting, or drumming ceremonies can evoke non-ordinary states of consciousness that facilitate healing at the level of the soul.

Recent advances in neuroimaging and affective neuroscience have illuminated how creative engagement restructures neural networks. When clients immerse themselves in art-making, sensors in their parietal lobe (responsible for spatial processing) and their limbic system (emotion regulation) often show increased coherence. This neural integration underlies expressive art therapy's reported mood-stabilizing and anxiety-reducing effects. Furthermore, art's repetitive, rhythmical aspects, such as brushstrokes or clay molding, can engage right-hemisphere processes associated with implicit memory and emotional regulation, creating a bridge to preverbal experiences stored deep in the brain.[2]

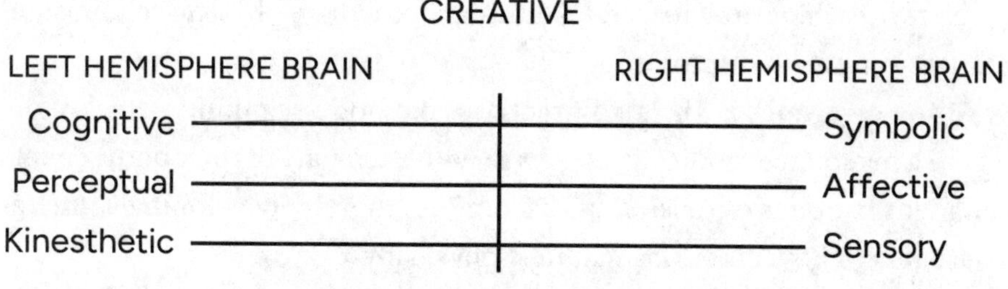

Figure 5. Expressive continuum

Expressive Therapies Continuum

The expressive therapies continuum delineates the different levels of functioning through which individuals interact with expressive arts, from raw sensory experience to symbolic cognitive processes. The continuum helps guide therapists' use of various expressive art modalities to support healing.

Level 1: Kinesthetic/Sensory

At the most fundamental level, the kinesthetic/sensory stage engages the body's primitive, preverbal processing systems. This stage is characterized by activities that stimulate the body's sensory and motor functions. For instance, engaging in rhythmic movement, tactile exploration through mediums like clay, or large-scale painting on canvases can activate the primal regions of the brain responsible for basic sensory feedback. This activation has several benefits:

Preverbal memory access: Many of our earliest experiences are stored nonverbally. We can reconnect with these early memories by engaging in activities that stimulate sensory awareness. Such reconnections can bring to the surface repressed emotions or sensations that may remain inaccessible in verbal therapy.

Calming effects: Kinesthetic activities often ground the nervous system. For example, rhythmic activities such as dancing or yoga can help regulate breathing and heart rate, offering immediate physical calming and reducing anxiety symptoms.

Body awareness: Through practices like body scanning, a technique where a person methodically checks in with each part of their body, clients can identify zones of tension or discomfort, thereby developing a greater awareness of how emotions manifest physically.[3]

Incorporating Stephen Porges's polyvagal theory adds depth to the kinesthetic/sensory stage. When clients engage in rhythmic movement or deep breathing, they activate the ventral vagal complex, fostering a state of safety that optimizes creative engagement. Therapists trained in polyvagal concepts can also recognize signs of a client's dorsal vagal shutdown and adapt their interventions, perhaps shifting to gentler sensory exploration before reintroducing more vigorous art-making.

Level 2: Perceptual/Affective

As clients progress from raw sensory experiences, they often move into the perceptual/affective level, where some verbal processing begins to merge with the expressive process. This stage is where the client begins to integrate their experiences, release emotions, and use the past as part of their expression:

Integration of experience: The creative process merges with cognitive functions, allowing individuals to attach meaning to their sensory experiences. Although the primary focus remains on expressing emotion, there is an emerging ability to name and label these emotions. This is a key step in transforming raw feelings into understandable experiences.

Emotional release: The perceptual/affective level focuses on the immediate experience of emotional release. Clients are encouraged to express feelings without worrying about the output's aesthetics. The emphasis is placed on the cathartic process of using art to externalize internal states.

Memory and narrative: Incorporating verbal elements into the creative process facilitates the integration of past experiences with present emotional states. Blending perception and affect can be potent for clients working through trauma, as it allows them to reframe painful memories within a safe, symbolic context.[4]

Level 3: Cognitive/Symbolic

The cognitive/symbolic level represents a more integrated stage in the expressive therapies' continuum. At this level, the creative process moves from being primarily somatic to engaging the full range of cognitive functions:

Symbolic expression: Creativity at this stage often involves using symbols and metaphors to represent complex issues. For instance, a client might use imagery or abstract forms to illustrate aspects of their identity or internal conflicts, making the abstract tangible.

Narrative construction: As cognitive functions become more involved, the therapeutic process incorporates a narrative dimension. Clients may construct stories or symbolic representations that articulate their journey, challenges, and insights. This narrative reflects their inner world and serves as a roadmap for healing.

Problem-solving: Integrating cognitive processing allows clients to approach their issues with a sense of problem-solving and agency. By externalizing internal conflicts through art, clients can observe their problems from a new perspective, leading to novel insights and solutions.[5]

At the cognitive/symbolic stage, exploring the metaphorical language clients create becomes an art. Therapists can introduce "metaphor mapping," in which a client's symbols are systematically unpacked, color by color, shape by shape, to reveal layers of meaning. This analytic approach complements the more free-form narrative construction.

Level 4: Creative

The final level, creative, is where the healing process reaches its most integrative and transformative potential. At this stage, all previous levels, kinesthetic/sensory, perceptual/affective, and cognitive/symbolic, are brought together in a dynamic synthesis: holistic expression. The creative level is about expressing, understanding, and integrating emotions.

Here, the client produces art that is a culmination of sensory experiences, emotional processing, and cognitive reflection. The work often transcends conventional boundaries, offering a comprehensive expression of the self.

The creative level offers a transformative potential that can inspire hope and empowerment. Here, clients can explore the full spectrum of their emotional and physical experiences. Holding and processing a wide array of feelings, from joy to sorrow, anger to peace, can be profoundly transformative. Clients learn that even the most difficult emotions can be experienced, expressed, and integrated into a broader healing narrative, which instills a sense of hope and inspiration about the healing journey.

Ultimately, reaching the creative level in expressive art therapy can empower clients by affirming their capacity to navigate and transcend personal challenges. The creative process becomes a tool for resilience, offering both a means of expression and a method for reimagining one's life narrative. Clients' self-empowerment can make them feel in control of their healing process and inspired to use their creativity as a tool for resilience.

Each level of the continuum can be subdivided to capture transitional moments. For instance, between the kinesthetic/sensory and perceptual/affective stages lies a "sensorimotor integration" sublevel, where clients notice patterns in their actions, such as repeatedly squeezing clay in order to mirror clenched anger. Recognizing these emergent patterns can accelerate insight.

Somatic Techniques with the Expressive Arts

When integrated with expressive arts, somatics strengthen the therapeutic process by directly engaging the mind–body system. This section explores six core somatic techniques: body scanning, trauma-informed breathwork, movement-based regulation, resourcing, therapeutic touch, and mindfulness-based somatic tracking, each of which supports clients in accessing embodied awareness and integrating emotional material.

All these techniques can interact with creative processes to support an embodied, culturally attuned, and accessible trauma recovery.

Body Scanning

Body scanning invites clients into a slow, deliberate survey of their internal landscape, identifying tension or numbness as invitations to deeper inquiry. Beyond the classic head-to-toe approach, advanced body scanning can integrate subtle variations to deepen interoceptive awareness. Instead of sweeping through broad regions, therapists can guide clients to focus on micro-zones, such as the front of the throat, the space between the shoulder blades, or the webs between their fingers. When clients isolate these smaller areas, even faint sensations (a slight warmth, a hint of tightness) become detectable. This granularity can reveal buried emotional residues that larger scans might overlook.

After identifying tension, clients are invited to pair that awareness with an expressive art gesture, such as tracing the sensation's silhouette with a charcoal stick on paper. This simultaneous scan-and-draw embeds bodily data into visual form, fostering a direct soma-graphic link between felt experience and artistic representation.

Incorporating gentle micro-movements, such as subtle head tilts, ankle rolls, or finger flexes, while scanning can help clients differentiate static tension from areas that release under motion. Observing where movement amplifies or diminishes tension deepens insight into how trauma or stress has become "stuck" in the musculoskeletal system.[6]

Trauma-Informed Breathwork and Resourcing

Breathwork is a powerful tool that enhances relaxation and facilitates emotional release. Techniques such as deep diaphragmatic breathing help regulate the nervous system, reduce anxiety, and create a state of calm that can make the creative process more accessible and practical. Because breath-focused practices can sometimes evoke activation, they are paired with resourcing strategies that help clients locate internal and external supports. Resourcing may involve visualizing a safe space, recalling supportive memories, or identifying tangible sources of comfort in the environment. By establishing this foundation of safety, clients can engage in breathwork without becoming overwhelmed.

Screening, safety, and preparation: Before beginning any new breathwork practice, therapists must conduct a thorough pre-session screening, which ensures client safety and readiness. This process starts with a detailed medical and respiratory history intake, where the therapist inquires about any diagnoses such as asthma, chronic obstructive pulmonary disease, cardiovascular conditions, or vertigo that could be exacerbated by breathwork. In parallel, a trauma sensitivity assessment helps identify any dissociative tendencies or past panic responses associated with breath-focused interventions. Understanding whether the client's previous breathwork experiences were neutral, beneficial, or distressing allows the therapist to tailor the session accordingly. Finally, co-creating a grounding plan with the client, comprising two or three personalized anchors like a comforting object, an evocative image, or a soothing phrase, lays the foundation for safety. Practicing these anchors briefly in session ensures that clients can shift into a self-soothing state swiftly should distress arise during breathwork.

Breath awareness practices: Therapists can introduce clients to breath-focused attention that does not alter their natural respiratory patterns. The therapist invites the client to observe the rise and fall of their body for one to two minutes, encouraging a soft focus on sensations at their nostrils or abdomen. There is no instruction to change how they breathe; the goal is simple awareness of their breath's inherent rhythm. The next step, micro-breath pausing, gently expands this awareness by asking the client to hold briefly, approximately one second, after each exhalation, only if it feels comfortable. Over five to eight cycles, the therapist checks in on the client's experience, to ensure that any sensation of discomfort immediately releases the hold. After the client completes a set of micro-breaths, the session pauses for a resourcing check-in: The client is invited to activate their previously practiced anchor, whether by holding their chosen object, visualizing their safe image, or repeating their grounding phrase. This alternation of micro-breath practice and anchor activation familiarizes the client with shifting between breath awareness and safety resources, building confidence that they remain held and supported.

Diaphragmatic breathing: Once clients demonstrate comfort by observing their breath, stage two introduces gentle support to encourage diaphragmatic expansion. The client places one hand on their lower ribs or abdomen, ideally atop a small bolster or folded blanket positioned beneath the ribs for tactile feedback. As they inhale, they are guided to feel a gentle outward push against their hand or the prop; as they exhale, they notice the softening and sinking of the hand. The therapist counts two to three seconds for each inhalation and exhalation, and reminds the client that these durations are flexible and can be shortened if they become uncomfortable. The presence of the bolster provides somatic verification of actual belly breathing, while the counted rhythm offers a shared structure. The therapist pauses the exercise every three to four breath cycles to facilitate a brief resourcing integration: The client notes any shifts in bodily or emotional tone and re-engages their grounding anchor as needed. This repeated alternation between supported breathing and resource activation deepens diaphragmatic awareness while maintaining a continuous safety net.

Rhythmic breathing and creative integration: Clients then build upon diaphragmatic practice by weaving in gentle rhythmic continuity and opportunities for creative visualization. They pace their breath at approximately three seconds for inhalation, imagining drawing in a chosen "resource" color, and three seconds for exhalation, imagining releasing a "tension" color. While breathing, the client traces a simple arc or circle on paper, allowing the visual line to mirror their breath cycle. After five complete breath-draw cycles, the therapist offers an expressive prompt such as "Sketch the shape your breath made" or "Write one word that arose." These short art-making breaks reset the client's attention, preventing cognitive overload and allowing insights to emerge organically. Titration remains central. Therapists should feel patient and understand the gradual progression in this stage, as it ensures the client's comfort and stability.

Advanced breathwork and expressive expansion: For clients who have consistently demonstrated stability and comfort in earlier stages, therapists can offer deeper breathwork patterns. One option is box breathing paired with art response: The client inhales for four seconds, holds for two, exhales for four, and holds again for two, then spends thirty seconds sketching any emergent image or emotion. Alternating between contained breathwork and rapid creative expression deepens the mind-body connection. For those ready for more intense experiences, the therapist can incorporate a tentative holotropic-inspired cycle, brief rapid breathing at a one-to-one ratio for one to two minutes. Immediately following this accelerated sequence, the client collapses into a pre-prepared art station (clay, charcoal, acrylics) and allows spontaneous imagery to flow. Throughout these deeper interventions, the therapist remains within arm's reach; grounding objects and personalized anchors are at hand, with an exit cue (such as three taps) agreed upon in advance. Hence, the client retains full agency over pacing and intensity.

Daily engagement: After each breathwork session, integration practices help the client consolidate gains and foster daily engagement. They begin with a two- to three-minute grounding routine that repeats the same steps used earlier, observing the natural breath while activating their chosen anchor. Then the client completes a breath journal entry, noting which stage they practiced, any noticeable bodily or emotional shifts, and a quick doodle or keyword that captures that moment. The therapist also instructs them to return to micro-breaths and their anchor in their at-home practice if breathwork ever feels activating. These integration steps empower the client to bring the session's safety framework into everyday life, reinforcing that they can self-regulate and creatively express at any moment.[7]

Movement-Based Regulation

For many individuals, movement is an effective mode of both regulation and expression, especially when words are insufficient. Dance and other forms of movement therapy allow clients to embody their emotions, releasing tension and expressing feelings that might be too complex or painful to articulate verbally. Movement can serve as a metaphor for change, symbolizing the fluidity and evolution of the self.

Safety and grounding: Before initiating any movement-based intervention, therapists must conduct a thorough screening and preparatory process to establish both physical and emotional safety. The therapist begins by reviewing the client's medical history, paying particular attention to musculoskeletal issues, vestibular or balance concerns, and any cardiovascular or respiratory limitations that could be aggravated by movement. Concurrently, a trauma history intake assesses the client's past somatic triggers, such as flashbacks during exertion or sensations of helplessness in the body, that might arise once movement begins. Together, therapist and client co-create a movement safety plan designed to provide the client with personalized grounding anchors, such as a specific hand gesture, a soothing phrase, or a small tactile object, to use in case of overwhelming sensations during movement exercises. This plan is a crucial part of the therapeutic process, as it ensures the client's safety and helps them feel more in control during the sessions.

From micro-movements to supportive exploration: A therapist gently introduces movement as simple invitations rather than directives. The client is guided to notice spontaneous shifts in posture or breath as they stand or sit with eyes closed, simply acknowledging any impulses to sway, stretch, or adjust. Without imposing structure, the therapist names these micro-movements, "I see your shoulder tilting, your hip releasing," thereby validating the body's innate wisdom. Next, the client explores tiny, localized movements, such as finger flexes, ankle rolls, or gentle shrug-and-release sequences, never exceeding a safe range. After each brief micro-movement set, sessions pause for a grounding check-in: The client activates one of their anchors, rooting themselves in stability before proceeding. Oscillating between movement and resourcing cultivates trust in their body and reinforces that agency lies at the client's fingertips.

Once clients demonstrate comfort with micro-movements, the protocol shifts to supported exploration of broader movement patterns. In this stage, the therapist's role is to guide and support the client as they experiment with simple gestures, such as raising their arms overhead on an in-breath and lowering them to the heart center on an out-breath, while maintaining gentle contact with a wall or sturdy chair for balance. The therapist may also introduce props like scarves, ribbons, or lightweight balls to extend movement through space without demanding full weight-bearing. Breathing remains central, and the therapist cues a slow rhythm to avoid hyperventilation, customizing inhalation and exhalation counts to the client's lung capacity. Following each supported sequence, the client revisits their grounding anchor and is invited to sketch a quick line or shape on paper that mirrors how the movement felt, linking somatic experience to creative expression.

Melding expressive arts and movement: Movement and expressive arts converge in longer, more fluid sequences that honor the client's emerging somatic narratives. Integrative expressive movement is designed to help clients express their feelings and experiences through movement and art. To accompany movement, a client can choose one or two art materials, such as watercolor on floor-spread paper or soft clay on a low table. As they flow through a gentle torso twist, they might drip pigment from a brush held in each hand, allowing color to mark the trajectory of their body. The therapist emphasizes the primacy of felt experience over aesthetic outcome, reminding the client that "every smudge, every arc is a word your body wants you to hear." Between movement-art segments, the client pauses to activate their grounding anchor, reflect on any sensations or images that emerged, and note one word or doodle in a movement journal. This cyclical integration ensures that intensifying movement remains tethered to safety resources and creative meaning-making.

Expansive improvisation and somatic expression: For clients who have demonstrated stable regulation and clear embodiment of earlier stages, therapists can offer expansive, improvisational movement-expression. In a spacious area, the client may engage in undirected "movement dialogues" with the therapist or with recorded music that shifts in tempo and tone. They might use floor-painting techniques, walking through diluted paints on large sheets of paper, to trace personal pathways or thresholds. Touch can be introduced here as a self-applied massage with aromatic oils, encouraging clients to notice how movement and touch modulate emotional release. Throughout these advanced exercises, the pre-negotiated exit cues and grounding anchors remain immediately available, and the therapist remains attuned to subtle shifts that signal overstimulation, ready to guide the client back to micro-movements gently if needed.[8]

Therapeutic Touch and Mindfulness-Based Somatic Tracking

Touch techniques, such as massage therapy, Reiki, or other bodywork practices, can be instrumental in processing emotions stored in the body. When integrated with expressive arts, touch can help bridge the gap between the physical and emotional realms, facilitating deeper release and healing. Touch bodywork is not done by the therapist but by a qualified, licensed, certified professional who can collaborate with the client and the therapist.

Mindfulness-based somatic tracking weaves attention, sensation, and present-moment awareness into a stable foundation for expressive work. Mindfulness and meditation practices also encourage clients to develop a heightened awareness of bodily sensations and emotions. Meditation techniques can help ground their mind and body, allowing clients to observe their inner experiences without judgment. This non-reactive awareness is crucial for creating a safe space for healing.

Guiding the Creative Healing Process

In expressive art and somatic therapies, the therapist serves as both facilitator and co-creator in the healing process. Their role centers on cultivating a physically, emotionally, and culturally safe environment through clear boundaries, creative choice, and attunement to the client's needs. While the client is the primary artist, the therapist guides the process, offering structure, validation, and interpretation of symbolic expression, to help transform their raw creativity into insight and integration. By affirming clients' autonomy and innate capacity for self-healing, therapists support them in reclaiming their agency and resilience.

Creative expression is a universal language, so therapists can tailor their approaches to fit each client's unique cultural and personal contexts. Therapists must understand that expressions of art and somatic experiences can vary widely across cultural backgrounds. For example, clients with a history of trauma require a delicate approach. Therapists must recognize that specific modalities, especially those involving physical touch or movement, might trigger past traumatic experiences. A trauma-informed approach involves carefully assessing what techniques are appropriate and modifying interventions to ensure the client feels safe and supported. Clients from marginalized or oppressed backgrounds may have unique experiences and challenges deeply intertwined with their identities. Expressive art therapy can be an exceptionally potent tool for these individuals, allowing them to express their lived experiences and reclaim their narratives in a validating space. Every client comes with their own preferences, experiences, and healing needs. Therapists must continually assess the client's comfort level with various techniques and adapt their approach based on the client's feedback and observed responses. What works well for one individual may be too overwhelming for another.

The field continues to evolve, informed by neuroscience, psychology, and cultural studies. Insights into neuroplasticity underscore the power of creative expression to reorganize neural pathways, fostering emotional regulation and adaptive responses to stress and trauma. With the emergence of digital art forms, therapists can expand traditional practices into immersive, technology-enhanced modalities that personalize the therapeutic experience.[9]

Expressive art therapy now extends beyond individual practice to include community art initiatives and group workshops that nurture connection and collective healing. These approaches highlight creativity's vital role in building resilient communities and addressing social injustice and collective trauma.[10]

By engaging body, mind, and spirit through art-making, movement, breathwork, and mindfulness, therapists help clients reconnect with themselves and integrate fragmented experiences into new narratives. In doing so, expressive art therapy stands as a testament to human resilience, reminding us that healing is both deeply personal and profoundly creative.

Case Example: Using the Expressive Continuum

Expressive art therapy offers a framework for working with clients whose emotional processing and self-regulation have been affected by various life challenges. In this case, the client was a teenage cis-gender woman (she/her) nearing her eighteenth birthday. She identified as white and bisexual and came from a lower-income background. She struggled significantly with emotional regulation after experiencing bullying due to her sexual orientation. This case example is an ideal lens to examine the integration of the expressive continuum and somatic approaches within art therapy. In the following sections, we will explore the clinical reasoning behind the interventions, detail the step-by-step processes used, and situate the work within broader theoretical and cultural contexts.

The client's challenges included emotional dysregulation. She faced a constant barrage of negative experiences at school that led to an overwhelming sense of emotional dysregulation. She experienced difficulty managing the physiological responses triggered by repeated trauma. Negative internal narratives, such as bullying, often leave deep-seated internalized messages. In this case, the client had internalized negative labels and associations related to her body and identity, which hindered her ability to process her experiences. She felt somatic distress because the body carried the memory of her emotional pain, manifesting in tension and dysregulation. This was evident in the way her body reacted to discussions of her identity and experiences of rejection. Finally, she struggled with self-expression, as traditional talk therapy had not provided sufficient relief from her symptoms. Her physiological responses persisted, which made it difficult for her to fully engage in verbal processing. She needed a more embodied approach that could bridge the gap between what she felt and what she could express.

The therapeutic journey with this client was conceptualized as a progression through the levels of the expressive continuum, each building on the previous one to support her growing capacity for self-regulation and narrative reconstruction. Given the client's intense physiological responses, characterized by a freeze or fight-flight reaction, initiating therapy with kinesthetic and sensory experiences was essential. Movement-based interventions serve to ground clients in the present moment and establish a sense of bodily autonomy. Clients whose nervous systems have been hijacked by trauma need grounding before they can do any cognitive processing.

One of the first techniques we employed was bilateral drawing. I invited the client to stand or sit comfortably and provided her with two charcoal pencils and a large sheet of paper. She created concentric circles simultaneously with both hands, an activity that served multiple functions, including regulating the nervous system by using both hands in a rhythmic pattern, which helped calm her nervous system. The bilateral nature of the activity facilitated cross-hemispheric integration in her brain, which is crucial for emotional regulation. The physical drawing allowed her to remain present in her body. The repetition and symmetry of the concentric circles acted as a meditative focus, redirecting her attention away from distressing internal narratives. Activating her kinesthetic memory by engaging in a structured and rhythmic movement, the client began to reconnect with the inherent wisdom of her body, a critical step in accessing and processing early, preverbal memories.

Sensory interventions such as bilateral drawing (see Figure 6) function as a means to access and modulate the physiological states that underlie emotional experiences. I remained attuned to the client's body language and subtle cues throughout, offering gentle guidance and validation. My

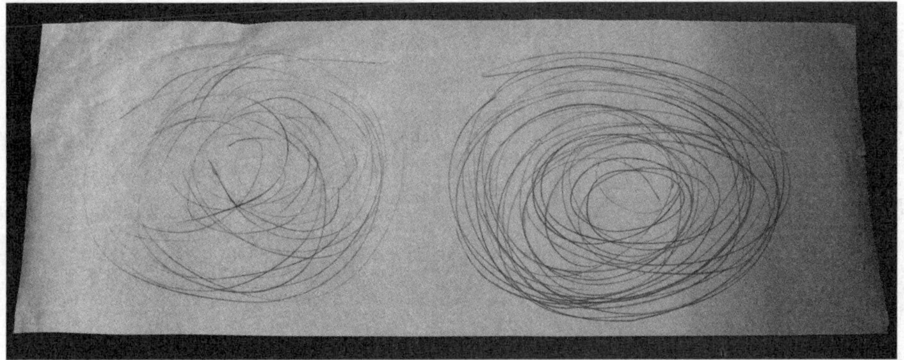

Figure 6. Bilateral drawing

role was to create a safe space where the client could experience a sense of agency over her bodily responses. Once she began to experience some degree of bodily regulation, the therapeutic process moved toward integrating perceptual and affective components. This transition opens the door to begin labeling and processing the raw emotions initially accessed through kinesthetic work.

At this stage, I introduced concrete studio art techniques, which allowed the client to explore her internal landscape visually. For instance, I encouraged her to experiment with painting in a controlled environment, emphasizing expression rather than perfection. With its fluidity and capacity for blending, the paint medium became a metaphor for the client's evolving emotional state. She was invited to select colors that resonated with her emotional experience. As she moved the brush across the canvas, the blending and overlapping of colors represented her internal world's complex, layered nature. I introduced elements of Gestalt therapy and drama to facilitate her emotional expression further. Through role-playing and enactment, the client could experiment with different facets of her identity, externalizing internal conflicts and imagining new, empowering narratives. These exercises provided a bridge between the raw sensory data of the kinesthetic and the more reflective processes that would follow. The transformative power of the therapeutic process was evident as she began to reconstruct her narrative, gaining a new perspective on her experiences and identity.

Integrating music into the therapeutic process was another key component of the perceptual/affective level. Music without lyrics, such as classical, was chosen specifically for its ability to evoke deep emotional responses without the interference of explicit verbal meaning. The client was invited to listen to selected pieces of music while engaging in painting. The auditory stimuli helped create an atmosphere of safety and openness so her emotions could surface organically, allowing for a stronger emotional connection. I encouraged the client to use the unfolding story of the music as a backdrop for her creative process. This process allowed her to draw parallels between the ebb and flow of musical notes and the rhythms of her own emotional experience. (It's important to note, however, that not all clients may respond positively to an integration of sound and image. Some may find it overwhelming or triggering. Adjusting the therapeutic approach and providing additional support are crucial in such cases.) Over time, the integration of sound and image enabled her to form a multisensory narrative of her journey that captured the turbulence and the beauty inherent in her identity.[11] The client's growing capacity for self-regulation was a testament to the effectiveness of the therapeutic process, encouraging both the client and the therapist to continue their work.

As the client's nervous system became more regulated and she felt more confident expressing herself through sensory modalities, the therapeutic process naturally progressed into the cognitive and symbolic domains. Her readiness for this stage was marked by her ability to reflect on and articulate the experiences she previously processed at a nonverbal level. At the cognitive/symbolic level, she was encouraged to create artwork representing the deeper meanings of her experiences. The creative process was no longer merely about sensory regulation or emotional release; it became a deliberate act of constructing a personal narrative.

I guided her to explore and represent her identity through symbols and metaphors. For instance, she could create an image that symbolizes the dual nature of her experience as a Queer individual, capturing both the fear of rejection and the joy of authenticity. Through symbolic representation, she was able to externalize and critically examine the labels and associations attached to her body. The therapeutic aim was to help the client neutralize the negative connotations attached to her identity. By reimagining her narrative through art, she could begin to see herself not as a victim of bullying and social marginalization but as a resilient individual capable of self-determination and transformation. This process of narrative liberation is central to many contemporary approaches in expressive art therapy, especially within the context of Queer identity work.

Combining cognitive knowledge with somatic experiences often creates what might be described as a "system override" in trauma therapy: The trauma response may still be present, but the client has learned to engage in reasoning and coping strategies that "override" it and provide them an alternative way of processing distress. In this case, I encouraged the client to reflect on her artwork and articulate the associations and feelings that emerged during the creative process. This reflective dialogue helped bridge the gap between her sensory and cognitive realms, facilitating a deeper understanding of how her body and mind interacted. By connecting the dots between her physical sensations, emotional expressions, and cognitive insights, she began to build resilience. Naming and contextualizing her feelings allowed her to challenge automatic responses and reframe her narrative. She felt empowered to view her identity through strength and possibility rather than fear and shame.

The final cognitive integration involved crafting a coherent narrative that unified the client's experiences. Storytelling became a central component of the therapy, providing a way to document her journey and affirm her evolving sense of self. Initially, her story was embedded in the visceral, nonverbal experiences of movement and sensory exploration. But as she gained greater cognitive insight, these experiences were transformed into a more deliberate narrative. This narrative was not a recounting of events but an active re-authoring of her identity, a process of liberation from the negative internalized messages imposed by bullying. The narrative work allowed her to explore existential questions such as *Who am I beyond the labels and the pain?* and *What does it mean to embrace my Queerness in a world that often misunderstands it*? Through guided reflection, journaling, and artistic expression, the client began to reconstruct her self-concept, embracing both the joy and the fear that coexist in her lived experience.[12]

Her narrative had been strongly affected by bullying and its effects. Bullying, especially when it targets one's sexual orientation, can inflict deep psychological wounds. In her case, the relentless taunts and exclusion at school not only undermined her sense of self but also contributed to a pervasive state of hypervigilance and fear. Such experiences often lead to internalized shame. Negative societal messages about Queer identities can also become internalized, leading to a diminished self-concept and feelings of unworthiness. The bullying had left her with internalized labels and a pervasive fear of rejection, which hindered her ability to express her true self. Her body bore the brunt of her emotional distress in the form of chronic tension, dysregulation, and a sense of disconnection from her physical self. This disembodiment further complicated her ability to process and integrate her experiences. She also dealt with a fragmented narrative, which happens when identity is attacked. Her story was split between the internalized messages of shame and the raw, authentic experience of her Queer identity; the therapeutic process aimed to reunify these fragmented parts into a coherent narrative of resilience and self-acceptance.[13]

As the client's story became clearer and her ability to regulate emotions improved, the choice of art materials gained increasing clinical importance. In guiding this next stage of her therapy, I used the medium dimension variable continuum to make sure each artistic choice supported her emerging therapeutic goals. The continuum shows how different media and processes can either anchor a client in sensory experience or encourage more symbolic, reflective engagement, depending on their readiness and needs. Therapists can strategically pick art media to help move along these processing levels, from the raw kinesthetic to the perceptual, emotional, and eventually cognitive stages. The continuum organizes art media based on several key properties (see Figure 7).

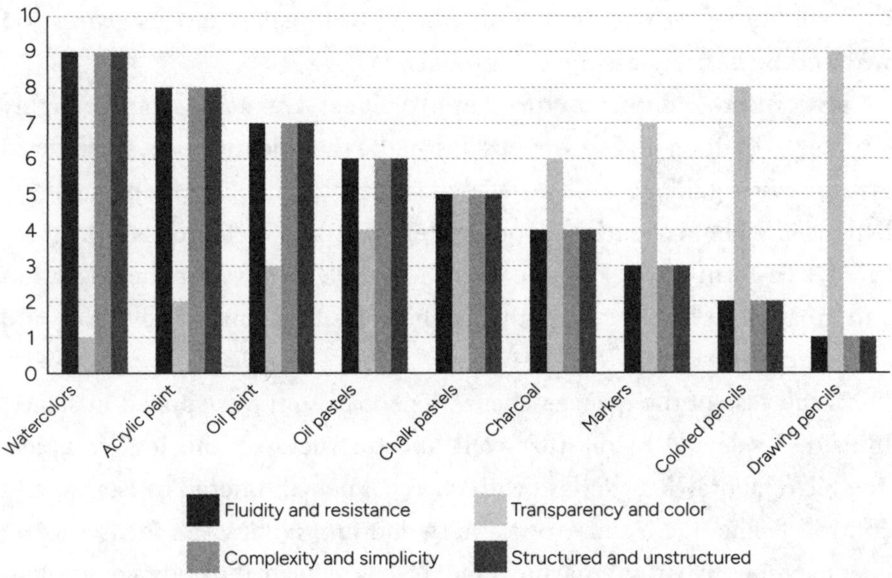

Figure 7. Medium dimension variable continuum

Fluidity and resistance: This dimension considers how malleable and controlled a medium is. For instance, watercolors are characterized by their fluidity and capacity for blending, which can evoke a sense of ease or unpredictability in emotional expression. In contrast, pencils and charcoal offer resistance and structure, lending themselves to more deliberate and controlled expressions. Clay is highly resistant and can be used to express deep-seated emotions. Pastels are fluid and can be used to create a sense of movement and change in the artwork.

Transparency and color: Here, the focus is on the opacity of a medium, as well as the vibrancy of its colors. Transparent media can symbolize vulnerability or the openness of one's internal state, while opaque, saturated colors may represent strength, intensity, or a bold desire to assert one's identity.

Complexity and simplicity: The skill level needed to manipulate a medium effectively is another key factor. Complex media require more artistic skill and control, which can serve as both a challenge and an opportunity for growth. Simpler media allow for spontaneous expression without the barrier of technical proficiency.[14]

Structured and unstructured approaches: Art-making can be highly structured or open-ended, depending on the therapeutic goals. Structured tasks provide guidance and a sense of security, which can be particularly beneficial when a client's nervous system is still in high arousal. Unstructured, free-form art-making, on the other hand, invites deeper exploration and creative risk-taking, supporting the transition toward cognitive and symbolic processing.[15]

In the case of the teenage client, the continuum was applied in stages. Initially, I selected media that were more structured and less complex. The bilateral drawing exercise with charcoal pencils offered resistance and control, facilitating a sense of stability and grounding. The focus was on creating repetitive, rhythmic movements that regulate the body's physiological response. As the client's regulation improved, I introduced more fluid media, such as watercolors, during painting sessions paired with classical music. The watercolors allowed her to explore the subtle interplay of emotions, capturing both the fluidity of her inner experience and the shifts in her emotional landscape. Combining structured and unstructured tasks helped connect the initial sensory regulation to the later stages of narrative construction. When she reached the cognitive/symbolic stage, the focus shifted toward media that supported more intentional and reflective work. By using mixed media, for example, she could combine elements of structure (through drawing or collage) with the spontaneity of painting or abstract art. This mix enabled a richer exploration of the symbols associated with her identity and the internalized narratives she was working to transform.

Finally, the therapeutic process culminated in sessions where the client was invited to select media that resonated most with her evolving narrative. In these sessions, the choices were made collaboratively, as I facilitated discussions about the meanings behind each medium's properties. This approach reinforced her autonomy and deepened her understanding of how the physical properties of art materials could mirror and influence her internal state.[16]

This case moved session by session, unlike previous case examples, with a more cumulative process. The first session was dedicated to establishing rapport and a sense of safety. Recognizing the client's vulnerability, I carefully explained the rationale behind the expressive continuum and the integration of somatic techniques. Emphasis was placed on the nonjudgmental therapeutic space, where every creative expression was valid. During the early interactions, I noted that the client exhibited signs of hyperarousal and a marked sensitivity to physical proximity and touch. These observations guided my decision to avoid techniques perceived as invasive or overwhelming. A simple bilateral drawing exercise gently introduced her to the process. It was engaging and was an immediate tool for regulating her nervous system.[17]

In subsequent sessions, the focus shifted to deepening the kinesthetic experience. The client was encouraged to experiment with different postures, standing, sitting, or even lying down, depending on what felt most natural and safe. Throughout the session, I guided her through a body scanning exercise, asking her to notice any tension or discomfort as she engaged in the drawing. We gently discussed these observations afterward to increase her body awareness. The bilateral drawing exercise evoked noticeable rhythmic patterns in her movement, which is associated with calming the freeze response, a common reaction in individuals who have experienced prolonged states of hyperarousal. I noted these shifts and reinforced the importance of rhythmic movement as a foundation for more profound work.[18]

From here, sessions transitioned to the perceptual and affective modalities by using studio art techniques to bridge the kinesthetic to visual expression. The sessions incorporated more concrete art techniques once the client could regulate her physical responses. I introduced a palette of paints and brushes, allowing her to transition from the structured movement of drawing to the fluid expression of painting.

During this session, I asked the client to choose colors that resonated with her emotions. The exercise was structured around the idea that each color and stroke could represent different facets of her inner experience.

As she moved her brush across the canvas, I encouraged her to reflect on the sensations and memories that emerged with each color transition. Classical music (specifically Chopin) was playing to enhance emotional resonance further. This music, selected for its lack of lyrics and emotive quality, served as an auditory stimulus that helped connect her sensory and perceptual processes. The client reported feeling like the music was guiding her brushstrokes, adding another layer to her emotional narrative (see Figure 8).[19]

Building on the success of the painting exercise, I introduced elements of Gestalt therapy and drama. This session involved role-playing exercises

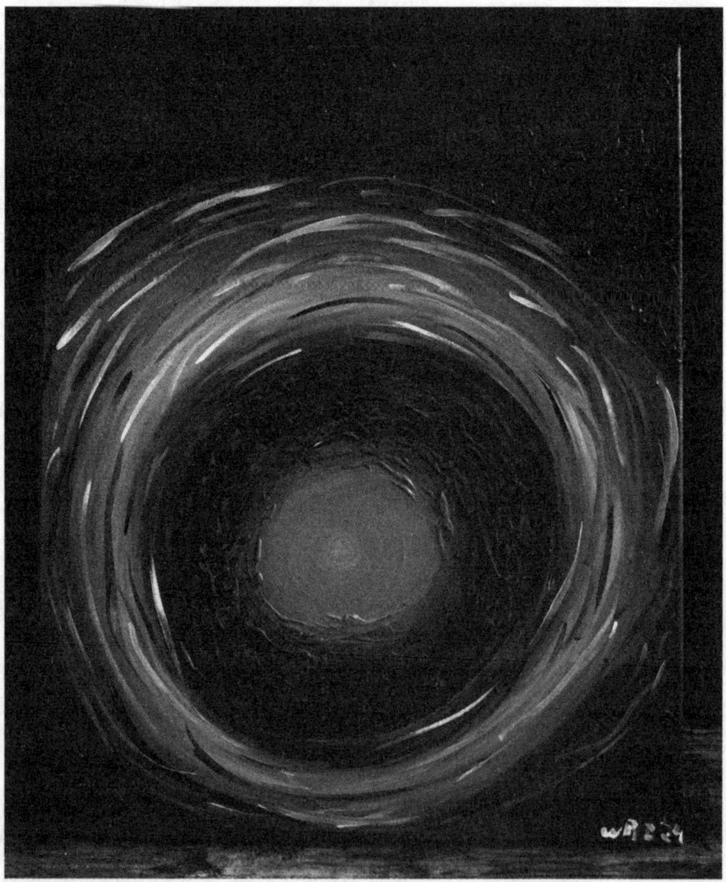

Figure 8. Music-inspired painting

that allowed the client to experiment with different expressions of her identity. For example, she was invited to portray various "selves," one who was burdened by internalized shame and another who embodied strength and resilience. By enacting different roles, she could externalize internal conflicts. As she shifted between roles, I observed changes in her posture, tone, and facial expressions, which were indicators of her internal emotional shifts. The process was cathartic, and she reported relief and empowerment after the session. Following the role-play, I asked the client to represent the experience visually. This exercise was designed to integrate her work's affective and perceptual components, using imagery to symbolize the conflict and eventual synthesis of her multiple identities.

As the client's ability to regulate her physiological responses improved, I introduced mixed media techniques. The client chose from various art supplies, from pencils and watercolors to collage materials. The aim was to encourage her to create layered artworks that symbolized the complex interplay of her emotions, body, and identity. During this session, she began articulating her associations with her body and identity. For example, specific images and symbols emerged that represented both the trauma of bullying and the resilience that was gradually taking shape within her. I worked with her to unpack these symbols, linking them to her lived experiences and the broader narrative of her self-discovery. The session concluded with a reflective dialogue. I invited her to discuss the meaning behind her artwork, exploring how specific colors, shapes, and symbols resonated with her internal world. This reflective process helped her integrate the somatic experiences of earlier sessions with a cognitive understanding of her journey.

At this stage, the therapeutic work focused on transforming fragmented experiences into a coherent narrative. I encouraged the client to create a series of artworks that collectively told the story of her journey from pain to resilience. Each piece served as a chapter in her evolving narrative. Alongside the visual work, she was invited to engage in journaling. She wrote about her feelings before, during, and after each creative session, linking the emotional experiences evoked by the art to the broader story of her identity. The process of journaling helped her solidify the insights she gained during the art-making process. The narrative work was explicitly aimed at reconstructing a sense of self that was both empowered and authentic. The client began to see herself as a resilient individual with the capacity to transform her traumatic experiences into strength. The co-construction of this narrative was a key milestone in her therapeutic progress.

The client's evolving relationship with her body and identity became increasingly evident throughout therapy. I observed several key transformations, including her increased self-awareness, reduction in negative internalized messages, and enhanced narrative coherence. Through the integration of sensory, affective, and cognitive work, the client developed a heightened awareness of her bodily sensations and emotional responses. She became adept at identifying areas of tension and could articulate the connections between these physical sensations and her internal experiences. The process of neutralizing negative words and associations allowed her to detach from the internalized shame and fear that had long dictated her self-perception. She began to adopt a more balanced view of herself, acknowledging the pain of past experiences and the strength that emerged from them. As the therapy progressed, her narrative shifted from being fragmented and dominated by trauma to one that was cohesive and empowering. The act of re-authoring her story gave her a sense of control and autonomy over her identity.

The therapeutic techniques used in this case are significant for clients with intersecting marginalized identities. For many Queer individuals, their journey toward self-acceptance is complicated by societal stigma and internalized oppression. Integrating expressive art therapy with somatic practices offers a model that validates lived experience, fosters resilience, and encourages community and connection. By using creative modalities that resonate with the client's unique cultural and social context, therapists can provide a validating space where the complexities of Queer identity are acknowledged and celebrated. The process of narrative liberation and embodied self-expression is inherently empowering. It equips clients with practical tools for coping with future challenges and fostering long-term resilience. The techniques discussed in this case can be adapted for group settings, where shared creative experiences foster a sense of community among individuals who have similarly experienced marginalization. This collective healing process is an essential aspect of building supportive networks.

The long-term impact of integrating art therapy with somatic practices is unique and significant. Beyond the immediate regulatory benefits, this approach has lasting effects on how clients relate to their body, process trauma, and construct meaningful narratives. The interwoven work of kinesthetic, affective, and mental techniques supports a holistic transformation that endures beyond the therapy sessions. The ability to express oneself creatively, especially in the face of external invalidation, is a powerful act of defiance and self-affirmation. Clients learn that their creative expression is more than an outlet for pain; it is a means of reclaiming their identity and rewriting their story. The techniques learned in therapy become tools that clients can apply to manage stress, process emotions, and navigate complex interpersonal situations in the future. Integrating sensory regulation with cognitive reflection provides a robust framework for ongoing self-care.

The case of the teenage client illustrates the deep impact that creative expression can have on healing. For many individuals, particularly those who have faced rejection or internalized societal stigma, art offers a pathway to reclaiming their voice. Through creating, reflecting, and integrating, clients discover that the canvas of their lives is not fixed but can be continuously reimagined and rewritten. One of the most significant shifts I observed in this client was her renewed connection to her body. Initially, her physical responses to stress were overwhelming, but through guided somatic practices, she began to trust her body as a source of insight and strength. This reconnection was pivotal in her journey toward self-acceptance and empowerment. Choosing how to express herself through drawing, painting, or movement allowed her to reclaim control over her narrative.

This client's journey did not end with the conclusion of formal therapy sessions. The techniques and insights she gained through expressive art therapy are tools she can draw upon whenever she faces stress, uncertainty, or challenges related to her identity, for the rest of her life. She learned various strategies, from bilateral drawing for immediate regulation to reflective journaling for processing deeper emotional narratives. She now has flexible options for self-care that respect her autonomy and allow her to choose the modality best suited to her emotional state at any given moment. Perhaps the most significant outcome was the shift in her self-identity. No longer defined solely by the pain of bullying or the internalized shame of societal rejection, she began to see herself as a complex, resilient individual with a rich tapestry of experiences. The creative process facilitated this shift, by allowing her to explore and integrate multiple facets of her identity, both the vulnerable and the powerful.

This case example is a microcosm of the broader potential inherent in expressive art therapy. It highlights the necessity of a multi-level approach that addresses not only cognitive and emotional aspects but also the vital somatic experiences that underpin trauma and identity work. One of the key lessons is the importance of flexibility in therapeutic interventions. The progression from kinesthetic to cognitive levels is not linear; it must be adapted to each individual's pace, history, and current state. The case demonstrates that a sensitive, client-centered approach is essential for fostering meaningful change. Beyond individual healing, expressive art therapy has the potential to build bridges between isolated individuals and the larger community. Group interventions and community-based art projects can amplify the healing process, providing collective support and validation. For Queer communities and other marginalized groups, an opportunity to create shared narratives of resilience and empowerment can be a transformative experience.

For clients who have struggled with traditional talk therapy, especially those whose body continues to react to unresolved trauma, the expressive continuum offers a new way forward. It acknowledges the complexity of human experience and honors the multifaceted nature of identity. In doing so, it creates a space where the body's silent narrative can be heard, where pain can be transformed into beauty, and where the journey from distress to liberation is not only possible but deeply empowering.

Ultimately, the story of the teenage client is emblematic of a larger truth: that the path to self-acceptance and healing is as varied and unique as the art we create. The journey is marked by vulnerability, courage, and the transformative power of creativity. For those who have long suffered in silence, the language of art and movement offers a powerful means of reclaiming their narrative and the essence of who they are.

By weaving together kinesthetic regulation, perceptual exploration, cognitive processing, and narrative liberation, therapists can offer a holistic pathway to healing that respects the full spectrum of human experience. Whether working with Queer youth, trauma survivors, or anyone struggling with the weight of negative internalized narratives, this integrated approach provides the tools necessary to unlock the innate resilience and creative power within us all. Through the careful balance of art, movement, and narrative work, somatic and expressive art therapy transcends the limitations of traditional modalities to offer clients a vibrant, dynamic process of healing that is deeply personal and universally human.

PRACTICE EXAMPLE

Integrative Somatic and Creative Practice

In a safe, adaptable space, the therapist invites the client to begin by gently tuning in to their body, taking a few moments of diaphragmatic breathing, noticing where tension or ease resides in the chest, belly, or limbs, before reaching for two drawing tools (pens, charcoal, or markers) to make symmetrical, bilateral marks on paper, allowing rhythmic, mirrored circles or lines to emerge in tandem with the breath as a bridge between sensation and creativity.

Without pausing, the client is then encouraged to move fluidly into a tactile collage or painting phase: selecting papers, fabrics, or paints that resonate with current inner landscapes, whether that's a color that feels like safety or a texture that echoes tension, and layering these materials onto a larger surface while continuing to monitor bodily sensations, pausing as needed to name what arises ("warmth in my hands," "tightness in my throat") and using that awareness to guide each choice of color, stroke, or glue.

As imagery takes shape, ambient music without lyrics plays softly in the background to evoke emotional resonance, prompting the client to experiment with the tempo of their marks, slow and flowing or quick and staccato, so that sound, movement, and visual expression intertwine. Finally, the client steps back, places a hand over their heart, and speaks or journals a brief affirmation or insight inspired by the artwork ("I am allowed to feel safe," "My story is multidimensional"), thereby weaving somatic attunement and expressive creation into a cohesive practice that any individual can adapt to honor the body's wisdom and the transformative power of art.

4

Practicing Harm Reduction in Somatic and Expressive Art Therapies

Queer bodies carry histories, narratives, and experiences that are as diverse as they are resilient. Acknowledging the multiplicity of these experiences is essential in the context of therapeutic practices. Traditionally, therapy has been structured around norms that may not fully capture the lived realities of Queer individuals. Integrative approaches, specifically harm reduction, somatic therapy, and expressive art therapy, offer nuanced ways to work with the body, mind, and spirit. These modalities help create spaces that honor individual truths, foster self-expression, and support healing.

Harm reduction is grounded in pragmatic strategies that acknowledge the reality of risk behaviors and focus on minimizing harm rather than enforcing abstinence. Somatic therapies emphasize the body's importance in storing and processing trauma, recognizing that healing often requires a reconnection with bodily sensations and experiences. Expressive art therapy leverages creative processes, such as art, movement, music, and writing, to facilitate emotional exploration and healing. When used together, these approaches provide a robust framework for Queer individuals to navigate challenges, validate their experiences, and cultivate holistic well-being.[1]

Harm reduction strategies emerged from the lived experience of people who use substances and the gamut of experiences they had as a result of the sociopolitical structures surrounding the treatment of substance use and the people who use them. This was later adopted as a public health practice, acknowledging the limitations of punitive or abstinence-only models. Harm reduction is about meeting individuals where they are, recognizing and addressing different behaviors, and working collaboratively to reduce negative consequences. Rather than demanding behavioral change, this approach emphasizes safety, self-determination, and incremental progress based on the client's desires, not our own.

In the context of Queer populations, harm reduction can be especially important. Many Queer individuals face systemic discrimination, stigma, and trauma that complicate their relationship with their body and behavior. Integrating harm reduction into therapeutic practices means accepting that avoiding all harm is not the goal, nor is it possible; instead, the aim is to create supportive environments where Queer people can manage risk in ways that align with their values and circumstances. This empowerment is a key aspect of harm reduction that can instill confidence in therapists to support their clients effectively.[2]

The term "multiple truths" refers to the layers of identity and experience that Queer individuals embody. Queer bodies are not monolithic; they encompass a range of intersections, including race, class, gender expression, and cultural background. Each of these layers interacts with personal and societal narratives, often resulting in unique challenges and forms of resilience. Therapists working with Queer clients need to be aware of these challenges and resiliency in order to provide effective treatment.

By integrating harm reduction, somatic, and expressive arts therapies, therapists can address the complexity of Queer experiences. This approach honors both the external and internal landscapes of Queer bodies, creating a space where multiple truths can be acknowledged and integrated. For example, a Queer person who has experienced trauma related to their identity may benefit from a somatic approach to help process bodily sensations linked to that trauma. At the same time, expressive arts allow them to tell their story through metaphor, imagery, and creative exploration. Harm reduction, in turn, ensures that the strategies employed are compassionate and nonjudgmental, recognizing the realities of living in a society that can be hostile or invalidating. This commitment to creating affirming therapeutic environments is a key responsibility of therapists in supporting their clients' well-being.

Integrating harm reduction techniques into somatic therapy for Queer individuals involves an attuned understanding of how trauma, behaviors deemed "risky" by society, and resilience intersect in the body. Rather than pathologizing a client's behaviors or bodily responses, therapists using harm reduction frameworks validate the reasons behind these experiences. For instance, a Queer individual might engage in self-harming behaviors or substance use as a way of coping with internalized stigma or external rejection. A harm reduction approach does not immediately condemn these behaviors but instead seeks to minimize their harmful effects while validating the reasons behind them and exploring alternative coping methods. Within somatic work, this means paying close attention to how the body reacts to stress, trauma, or even the discussion of painful memories. Therapists can work with clients to identify safe practices that mitigate risk, for example, by incorporating grounding techniques or body-based mindfulness exercises. These interventions help clients remain present and connected to their body even when they are confronting distressing emotions.

Incorporating mindfulness practices in somatic therapy can help clients observe their bodily sensations without judgment. Mindful breathing exercises, body scans, and grounding techniques can support individuals in remaining present, reducing the likelihood of dissociation during therapy sessions. For Queer clients who have experienced trauma, mindfulness can serve as a bridge between their internal experiences and external realities. Gentle movement practices, such as yoga, tai chi, or even dance therapy, can allow people to explore bodily sensations in a safe, controlled manner. These modalities promote physical awareness, encourage self-expression, and help people reclaim bodily autonomy. For example, a therapist might invite a client to express a particular emotion through movement, transforming an abstract feeling into a tangible, embodied experience. In cases where trauma is significant, techniques like somatic experiencing allow for the gradual release of stored tension. Titration, slowly introducing and processing traumatic memories, ensures clients are not overwhelmed. When coupled with harm reduction, these techniques emphasize safety and self-regulation, providing a roadmap for healing that respects the client's pace and readiness. For instance, a somatic session might incorporate a check-in about the client's experiences with substance use or self-harm. The therapist can then work with the client to identify safer alternatives or adjustments that honor the client's need for expression and physical safety. This approach ensures that the therapeutic space is focused on healing and harm reduction, thereby promoting the client's overall well-being.

Expressive art therapy is a powerful complement to somatic work by giving voice to the experiences that may be felt in the body but are hard to articulate. For many Queer individuals, the process of identity formation and self-acceptance involves reconciling multiple, sometimes conflicting, narratives. Art can become a medium through which clients externalize and explore these narratives. The creative process can illuminate hidden layers of trauma, resilience, and desire through drawing, collage, dance, or music. Expressive arts can help clients map out their internal landscapes when integrated with somatic practices. For example, clients might visually represent their bodily sensations associated with a traumatic memory. This visual art becomes a tangible reminder of their experience, a form of embodiment transcending words. In this way, expressive arts facilitate self-expression and serve as a bridge to somatic awareness.

Integrating expressive arts with somatic and harm reduction approaches creates a holistic framework that acknowledges the full spectrum of human experience. While somatic therapies invite clients to tune in to their bodily sensations, expressive arts offer a creative outlet for processing and communicating these sensations. Harm reduction, in turn, ensures that this exploration is conducted safely, with an emphasis on reducing risk and supporting self-determination. For instance, consider a therapeutic session where a client begins with a grounding exercise to connect with their bodily sensations, followed by a guided movement where they express these sensations through dance. Afterward, the client might engage in a creative writing exercise, narrating the emotions and experiences that emerged during the movement. The therapist maintains a harm reduction framework throughout this process by checking the client's comfort levels, validating their experiences, and suggesting modifications as needed. This layered approach ensures that the client is exploring their inner landscape and doing so in a safe and empowering manner.

Queer individuals often have experiences of discrimination, invalidation, and marginalization that can create a significant amount of mistrust toward traditional therapeutic environments. Trauma, whether stemming from familial rejection, societal prejudice, or direct violence, can result in a disconnection from the body. When the body is perceived as a site of harm, reconnection through somatic work becomes both challenging and essential. Therapists who integrate harm reduction with somatic and expressive arts modalities must be particularly attuned to these issues. Establishing trust is paramount. Therapists should create explicitly affirming environments, recognizing that the client's experiences are valid and that the therapeutic space is a sanctuary from the hostile narratives they may encounter elsewhere. Therapists must be well-versed in the complexities of Queer identities and the historical contexts that shape their experiences. This includes understanding the intersections of race, gender, socioeconomic status, and cultural background. Training in cultural competence is not a luxury but necessary for providing effective and respectful care.

A core principle of harm reduction is creating a nonjudgmental space where clients feel safe expressing themselves without fear of repercussion. The therapist should be prepared to listen, validate, and collaborate with clients to identify practices that promote well-being. This can be as simple as asking open-ended questions about the client's comfort level with various interventions, or as complex as co-creating a personalized harm reduction plan that integrates somatic and creative modalities. Queer individuals often have had their autonomy undermined by societal structures, so treatment should empower clients by offering choices in their engagement with somatic practices and expressive arts. Whether the client prefers a slow, introspective exploration of bodily sensations or a more dynamic, creative process, the therapist's role is to facilitate that choice without imposing a predetermined path.

Building trust requires transparency about the therapeutic process. Therapists should clearly explain the rationale behind each modality and how they intersect. When clients understand the purpose behind exercises, whether harm reduction check-ins, movement practices, or creative writing prompts, they are more likely to engage fully and feel a sense of ownership over their healing journey. One of the inherent challenges in integrating these modalities is balancing the imperative of safety with the need for deep exploration. By nature, somatic and expressive arts therapies invite clients to venture into vulnerable emotional and physical territories. For many Queer individuals, these territories have historically been associated with pain or danger. Therefore, harm reduction is a central guiding principle. Therapists must remain vigilant to cues of overwhelm, ensuring that the exploration of trauma does not become re-traumatizing.

Given the diverse experiences of Queer individuals, flexibility is paramount. Therapists must tailor interventions to meet each client's unique needs. For some, gentle movement is sufficient to reconnect with their body, while others require a more gradual introduction to expressive arts. The harm reduction framework supports flexibility by recognizing that progress may be nonlinear and setbacks are part of the healing process. Queer individuals also navigate systemic barriers, such as discrimination in healthcare, social isolation, or economic challenges, that can complicate the therapeutic process. Therapists must recognize these external factors and be prepared to support clients in addressing broader issues by connecting them with community resources or advocacy groups that work on systemic change. In doing so, therapy becomes part of a more significant movement toward social justice and equity.

Emerging studies are beginning to document how harm reduction, somatic therapies, and expressive arts can synergistically promote healing.

As the body of evidence grows, it will be crucial for therapists to stay informed and adapt their practices based on the latest findings. A commitment to evidence-based practice enhances therapeutic outcomes and reinforces the legitimacy of these innovative approaches within broader mental health care systems. For integrative approaches to become more widespread, training programs for therapists must incorporate modules on harm reduction, somatic therapies, and expressive arts. Such interdisciplinary training would empower clinicians with the tools necessary to address the complexities of Queer experiences comprehensively.

The integration of harm reduction, somatic therapy, and expressive art therapy represents a transformative approach to supporting Queer bodies in their healing journeys. By acknowledging the multiple truths that Queer individuals embody, these modalities provide a holistic framework that honors both the physical and emotional dimensions of experience. Harm reduction principles ensure that the path to healing is marked by compassion, safety, and pragmatism, while somatic work reconnects clients with their bodily wisdom. In turn, expressive arts open avenues for creative self-expression, enabling individuals to articulate and integrate the myriad facets of their identity. This integrative approach is particularly potent for Queer individuals, who often navigate a complex landscape of internalized stigma, external discrimination, and historical trauma. By meeting clients where they are, providing flexible and adaptive interventions, and emphasizing empowerment and self-determination, therapists can help Queer individuals reclaim their narratives. In doing so, they foster individual healing and contribute to broader cultural shifts, transforming spaces of pain into arenas of possibility, resilience, and profound transformation.

Case Example: Using Harm Reduction in Somatic and Expressive Art Therapy

This case study illustrates the integration of harm reduction techniques with somatic and expressive art therapy for a client whose experiences of marginalization contributed to a range of mental health challenges. The client was a Black, asexual, non-binary individual in their forties (they/them) who has struggled with bulimia nervosa and post-traumatic stress disorder (PTSD) related to racism and transphobia experienced in a corporate work environment. Over the course of therapy, the client's long history of disordered eating behaviors and trauma symptoms has been intricately linked to the cumulative effects of microaggressions, overt discrimination, and hostile work dynamics. These factors have not only shaped the client's internal world but have also influenced how they experience and relate to their body within a society that frequently invalidates non-normative expressions of gender, sexuality, and race.

Recognizing the multifaceted nature of this pain, the therapeutic approach was designed to honor the client's intersecting identities while offering concrete tools to manage distress. Harm reduction was a guiding principle, ensuring that interventions respected the client's autonomy and prioritized safety. By integrating somatic techniques and expressive art therapy, I encouraged the client to explore their bodily sensations and internal narratives in ways that traditional talk therapy had not permitted.

This client has navigated a lifetime of intersecting oppressions. Being a Black, asexual, non-binary individual in a corporate setting has exposed them to multiple layers of discrimination. Their identity, while a source of personal strength, has also been misinterpreted and undermined by environments steeped in systemic racism and transphobia. As a result, the client developed disordered eating behaviors, specifically bulimia, as a maladaptive strategy to cope with the overwhelming stress, self-criticism, and internalized shame stemming from relentless invalidation.

In the workplace, the client experienced microaggressions on a regular basis. The subtle yet pernicious acts chipped away at their sense of self-worth. Overt acts of discrimination further compounded these effects, creating an environment where the client's identity was consistently devalued. This hostile atmosphere contributed to the onset of PTSD, where triggers related to past traumatic events would precipitate intense physiological and emotional responses.

The interplay of these experiences created a complex psychological landscape in which the client's body became both a repository of trauma and a battleground for reclaiming dignity. Within this context, I decided to utilize a multi-pronged therapeutic approach, incorporating harm reduction, somatic therapy, and expressive art therapy. Each modality addressed a specific facet of the client's struggles while reinforcing a holistic, embodied healing process.[3]

Harm reduction acknowledges that complete behavioral change may not be immediately feasible or even desirable for some clients. For this client, harm reduction was not solely about altering eating behaviors; it was also about mitigating the impact of trauma responses while validating the lived reality of their intersecting identities.[4] At its core, harm reduction emphasizes safety, autonomy, and incremental progress. It provides a framework for the client to make choices that reduce their immediate risks and increase their overall well-being. In practice, this means that interventions are carefully tailored to the client's current state, with a recognition that any positive shift, no matter how small, is a victory. By focusing on harm reduction, the therapeutic process respects the client's pace and acknowledges that healing is often nonlinear.[5] Within this framework, interventions are designed to create a buffer between the client and the triggers exacerbating their symptoms. For instance, harm reduction strategies involve identifying specific moments when eating disorder behaviors occur and collaboratively exploring safer alternatives.

The focus remained on reducing harm rather than enforcing rules, thus minimizing the risk of additional shame or self-judgment. In this case, I was guided by the understanding that harm reduction must be integrated with an appreciation for the client's embodied experience. By merging harm reduction with somatic and expressive art therapies, the intervention sought to address both the cognitive aspects of trauma and its physical and emotional manifestations.

For this client, whose trauma was inextricably linked to experiences of racism, transphobia, and workplace discrimination, the body had become a repository for pain as well as a source of resilience. I introduced somatic techniques, such as breathwork, movement, and body scanning, to help the client reconnect with their physical self and create a more integrated sense of identity. One of the primary somatic techniques utilized was breathwork. In early sessions, I guided the client through exercises emphasizing slow, deep breathing to regulate their nervous system. Focusing on the breath served as an anchor, grounding the client in the present moment and reducing the intensity of physiological responses triggered by traumatic memories.

In parallel with breathwork, I introduced gentle movement exercises. I recognized that the client's body often mirrored their internal state, characterized by tension and rigidity, so I encouraged experimentation with subtle movements. Whether it was a gentle sway while seated or a deliberate shift in posture, each movement was celebrated as a step toward reclaiming bodily autonomy. The process was intentionally gradual, and even the slightest change was recognized as valuable progress in building embodied awareness.

A pivotal component of the somatic approach was body scanning (see Figure 9). In these sessions, I led the client through guided meditations to identify tension, discomfort, or numbness. This practice was about developing a nonjudgmental awareness of their bodily sensations. Through this process, the client began recognizing physical tension patterns intimately connected to emotional distress.

For example, the client identified chronic tension in their shoulders and chest, areas that often correlated with feelings of vulnerability and exposure. By becoming aware of these sensations, the client could gradually articulate how these physical responses were linked to memories of discrimination and marginalization. This mapping of tension allowed for a more nuanced understanding of how trauma was "stored" in their body, providing a foundation for further healing work.[6]

In later sessions, the therapeutic process evolved to include self-soothing techniques as part of the somatic practice. The therapeutic relationship and approach demonstrated how gentle self-touch, such as placing a hand on the heart or softly massaging the shoulders, could be a

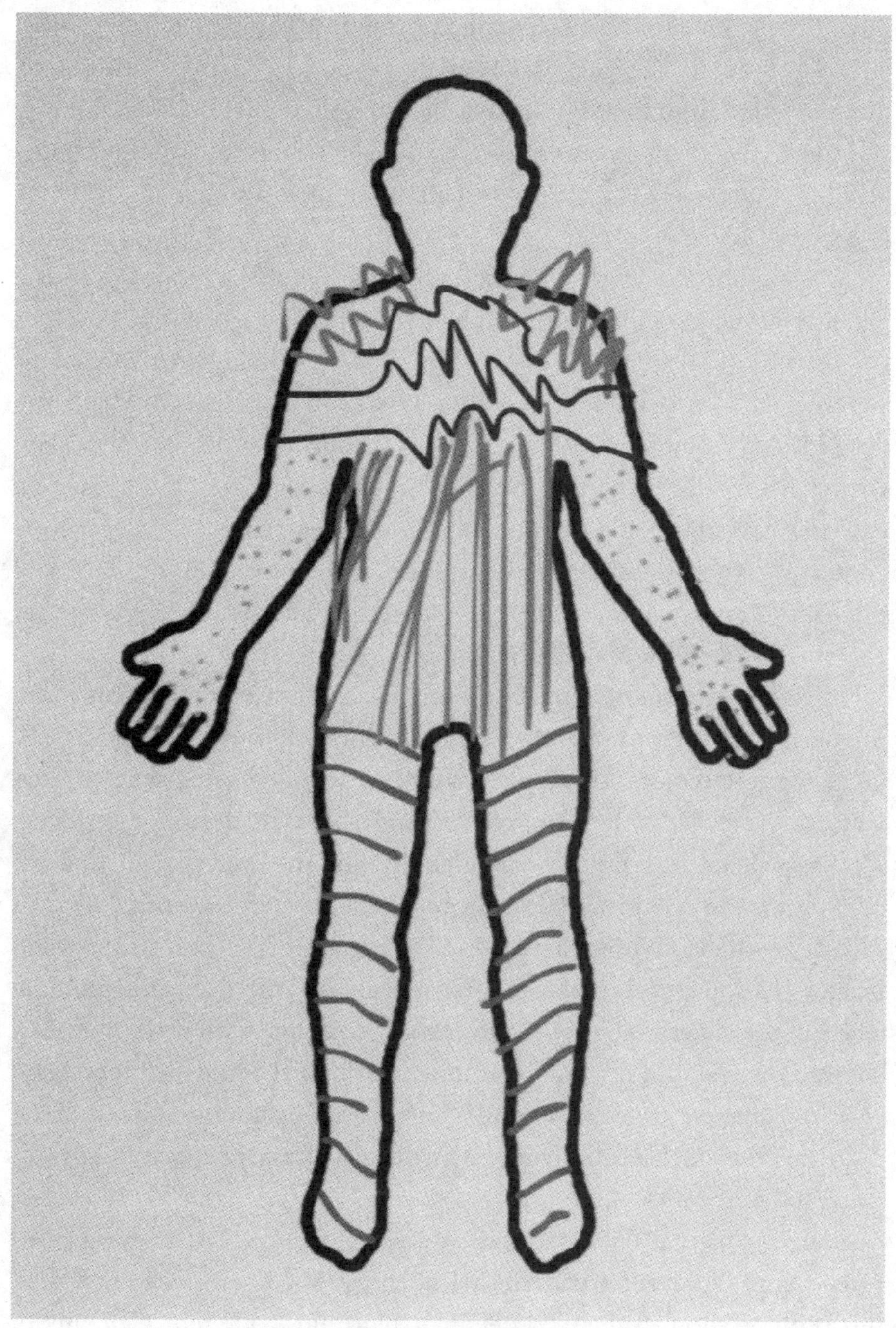

Figure 9. Chronic tension body scan

powerful reminder of care and self-compassion. This practice was particularly significant for the client, who had long experienced dissociation and a disconnection from their bodily self. By learning to offer comfort through self-touch, the client began to reframe their relationship with their body, viewing it not solely as a vessel for pain but also as a source of resilience and strength.

The gradual integration of these somatic practices empowered the client to develop a more compassionate internal dialogue. They began to see their body as an ally in the healing process, a living archive of their suffering and capacity for recovery. This shift in perspective laid the groundwork for integrating expressive art therapy into the treatment plan. Expressive art therapy gave the client a unique, nonverbal medium to explore, externalize, and reframe their internal narrative. In a therapeutic context where words alone were insufficient to capture the complexity of the client's experiences, art-making offered an alternative language that was as visceral as it was symbolic.[7]

In one of the foundational sessions focused on creative expression, the client was presented with a carefully curated array of art materials, including watercolors, charcoal, and collage supplies. We discussed each material in terms of its symbolic potential. Watercolors, for instance, were associated with fluidity, vulnerability, and the ever-changing nature of emotions. In contrast, charcoal embodied structure, contrast, and the capacity to mark out boundaries. With its layering of different textures and images, the collage was particularly significant in symbolizing the multiple facets of the client's identity. Choosing and engaging with these materials allowed the client to explore their inner world in a tactile and immediate way. The creative process became a form of self-exploration, inviting the client to confront painful memories while celebrating moments of resilience and possibility.

During a pivotal session, the client was invited to create an image representing the multiple truths of their identity. The open-ended nature of this prompt allowed them to deeply explore how different elements of their identity were interwoven with their experiences of trauma. As the

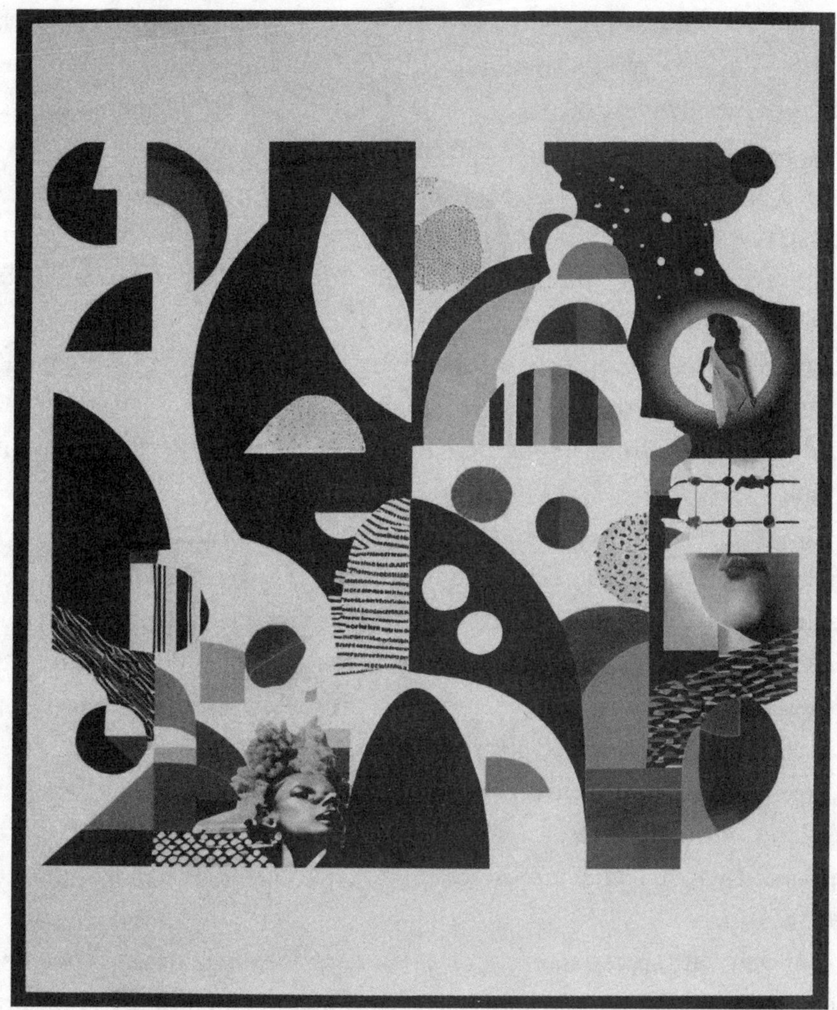

Figure 10. Multiple truths collage

client engaged with the materials, they began to layer images, colors, and textures to reflect the complexity of their internal experience. In a moment of creative breakthrough, the client produced a striking piece of art that juxtaposed stark contrasts. The artwork emerged as a layered collage that combined elements of darkness with vibrant bursts of color.

The phrase "multiple truths" not only signified the physical appearance of the artwork but also encapsulated the symbolic tension between pain and transformation. The stark black-and-white components reflect the persistent shadow of past traumas, while the vibrant splashes of color suggest hope, resilience, and the potential for renewal. In discussing the artwork, the client explained that the contrasts in the collage mirrored their internal struggle, where the pain of discrimination and marginalization coexisted with an emerging sense of self-empowerment and creative possibility. Expressive art therapy facilitated a dialogue between the client's inner experiences and the outside world. The creative process allowed the client to externalize conflicts that had long remained trapped in their subconscious. By putting these experiences into a tangible form, the client could view them from a new perspective, inviting reinterpretation and healing.

The session that produced the collage was a turning point. The client reported that engaging in creative expression allowed them to articulate previously indescribable feelings. Translating internal pain into visual imagery provided a powerful catharsis; the client could reclaim parts of their identity that had been suppressed by years of marginalization. I observed that the expressive art facilitated emotional release and served as a mirror for the client's evolving narrative. In subsequent sessions, the client returned to the artwork as a reference point, a reminder of the depths of their struggle and the resilience that had emerged through the creative process.[8]

Building on the collage's success, later sessions encouraged the client to explore their identity through various art forms. I introduced additional exercises, such as journaling alongside art-making and collaborative storytelling, to integrate the visual narrative with verbal expression. The client was invited to create a series of artworks over several sessions, each capturing different dimensions of their experience, moments of vulnerability, joy, and defiance in the face of systemic oppression. These exercises were particularly significant because they allowed the client to see their identity as multilayered and dynamic. The visual journal became a repository for the painful memories and the sparks of hope that punctuated their journey. Over time, the client's artwork gradually transformed: Images that once conveyed only pain evolved to incorporate self-compassion, empowerment, and renewal symbols. Integrating art into the therapeutic process underscored that healing is not a linear progression but a complex interplay of moments, emotions, and insights.

One of the most compelling aspects of this case study is the seamless integration of harm reduction with somatic and expressive art therapies. This integrative model was deliberately structured to support the client on multiple physical, emotional, and cognitive levels while respecting the client's autonomy and readiness for change. The very first session was dedicated to creating a secure, nonjudgmental space. Given the client's history of invalidation and marginalization, I needed to communicate a deep respect for their identity and experiences from the outset. We collaboratively established ground rules emphasizing confidentiality, informed consent, and the client's right to dictate the pace and content of the sessions. This initial stage laid the foundation for all subsequent work, ensuring that every intervention would be rooted in empathy and respect.

During this early stage, I introduced the core harm reduction concepts. Detailed discussions clarified that the focus was not on immediate cessation of disordered behaviors but on reducing harm and enhancing overall well-being. I encouraged the client to view any incremental progress as a success, a perspective that contrasted sharply with their previous experiences of rigid, all-or-nothing expectations.

With rapport established, the therapeutic process gradually introduced somatic interventions. In the second session, the focus shifted to grounding techniques designed to reconnect the client with their body. Recognizing that the client had experienced moments of dissociation and overwhelming physiological responses, I began with simple breathwork exercises. The client was invited to notice the inhaling and exhaling sensations, understanding that the breath could stabilize them during distress.

Gentle movement exercises were introduced to complement the breathwork. The client's rigid and disconnected physical posture often mirrored their internal state. In our work, I demonstrated that even the most minor adjustments could foster a sense of bodily ease by encouraging the client to experiment with slight movements, such as swaying or shifting weight while seated. This stage reinforced that harm reduction did not demand drastic changes; instead, it celebrated every small step toward a more embodied state of being.

As therapy progressed, sessions were dedicated to deepening the client's somatic awareness. Guided body scans where I led the client through systematic explorations of physical sensations became a recurring exercise. In one session, I asked the client to focus on areas where their tension was most pronounced, which often correspond to regions associated with traumatic memories. This practice allowed the client to map out how their stress and trauma were physically manifested, creating a bridge between internal emotional states and external physical sensations. I also introduced self-soothing techniques, one being gentle self-touch. Demonstrations on how to place a hand on one's heart or softly massage tense muscles provided the client with practical tools for self-regulation; this emphasis on self-care was significant, given the client's long-standing disconnection from their bodily self. Over time, the client began to report that these practices reduced their physical tension and fostered a renewed sense of trust in their body.

By the fifth session, the client was ready to embark on a process of narrative re-authoring, a collaborative exploration of the stories that had shaped their identity. Drawing on expressive art and somatic practices, the client was invited to reflect on their journey thus far. I structured the session around a dialogue that intertwined visual art with personal storytelling, emphasizing the notion of multiple truths in their narrative.

In this session, the client was asked to select a piece of their artwork that resonated most deeply with their evolving self-concept. The chosen piece served as a visual anchor, a reference point for discussing the interplay between past traumas and emergent strengths. As the client elaborated on the symbolism embedded in the artwork, I provided gentle guidance, ensuring the conversation remained within the client's comfort zone. Harm reduction principles were maintained throughout, and the client had the freedom to pause or shift focus if any aspect of the narrative exploration became overwhelming.

This collaborative narrative work marked a transformative stage in the therapeutic journey. The client began to articulate a re-authored narrative, one that acknowledged their wounds inflicted by racism, transphobia, and corporate oppression while simultaneously celebrating their resilience and creativity that had emerged despite these challenges. Integrating bodily awareness and artistic expression allowed the client to see themself not as a passive victim of circumstance but as an active agent in their healing and self-discovery.

In the final stage of this case study, the focus shifted to consolidation, integrating the progress made across sessions and establishing a roadmap for ongoing self-care and personal growth. The client and therapist revisited the tools and techniques developed throughout the therapeutic process. This "personal toolkit" from the client's journey encapsulated practices from harm reduction, somatic awareness, and expressive art therapy.

The consolidation session began with a comprehensive review of the client's progress. From their initial struggles with bulimia and PTSD to their gradual reawakening of embodied self-awareness and creative expression, their journey showed incremental yet meaningful transformations. We revisited key milestones in therapy, discussing how each intervention contributed to a deeper understanding of the self and the interplay between trauma and resilience.

In particular, the session highlighted the importance of harm reduction principles in the therapeutic process. I reminded the client that every small change, whether a more relaxed posture, a moment of mindful breathing, or the completion of a meaningful artwork, was a victory in its own right. The emphasis on incremental progress helped reframe the client's expectations, fostering an attitude of self-compassion and patience.

Looking forward, I collaborated with the client to develop a detailed self-care plan to sustain the gains they made during therapy. The plan included practical strategies for incorporating daily somatic practices, such as scheduled breathwork sessions, regular body scans, and periodic movement exercises. The client was encouraged to integrate these practices into their routine to maintain a stable connection with their bodily self. In parallel, expressive art was a continuing outlet for emotional processing and creative self-expression. The client committed to maintaining a visual journal, documenting their creative endeavors and the emotional insights that emerged from them. They envisioned the journal as a living document that could serve as a touchstone during moments of distress and as a reminder of the transformative journey unfolding throughout therapy.

The harm reduction framework was woven into the self-care plan. With my guidance, the client identified potential triggers for disordered behaviors and developed strategies to address these moments without resorting to punitive or rigid rules. For example, the client learned to recognize their signs of distress and engage in preemptive self-soothing practices rather than wait for the disordered behavior to escalate. This proactive approach underscored the harm reduction philosophy, emphasizing safety, autonomy, and continuous, incremental progress.

The consolidation stage also addressed the importance of external support networks. Given the client's experiences of marginalization in professional settings, engaging with supportive communities would be a critical component of long-term healing. We discussed various options including joining groups focused on Queer identity, art therapy communities, and local support groups that shared similar experiences of systemic oppression. These communities could provide ongoing validation and be places to share creative expressions and practice self-care strategies.

One of the most transformative outcomes I observed in this case was the client's gradual shift from a narrative defined by victimhood to one that spoke of empowerment and self-compassion. Initially, the client's identity had been overshadowed by the weight of past traumas and the invalidation they experienced in corporate and societal contexts. But they were able to re-author their story through the combined modalities of harm reduction, somatic awareness, and creative expression. The therapeutic process let the client externalize their internal conflicts, and ultimately enabled them to see themself as a survivor, a pearl that transformed pain into a source of strength.

Somatic therapy played a pivotal role in this transformation. The client could develop a more integrated sense of self by fostering an acute awareness of their bodily sensations and how trauma was "stored" in their body. The techniques of breathwork, movement, and body scanning were tools for immediate regulation that bridged the physical and emotional realms, and over time the client reported a newfound appreciation for their body's wisdom. Expressive art therapy provided a vital nonverbal outlet for exploring and reconfiguring their internal narrative. Creating the vibrant black-and-white collage (Figure 10) was a watershed moment in the therapeutic process, symbolizing the enduring impact of past traumas and the hopeful emergence of a reimagined identity. Through art-making, the client could visually manifest the complex interplay of emotions, experiences, and facets of identity that had long been silenced. This creative expression validated their experiences and reminded them of their capacity for renewal.

In this case example, the combined modalities enabled a Black, asexual, non-binary client in their forties to navigate complex issues surrounding bulimia, PTSD, and identity. By prioritizing safety, autonomy, and the body's inherent wisdom, the therapeutic process honored the multiple truths that the client holds, transforming pain into resilience and fostering a deep sense of self-empowerment.

The expanded narrative in this case study reveals that healing is a dynamic interplay of body, mind, and creativity. Each session, from establishing a secure, nonjudgmental space through the introduction and deepening of somatic practices to the transformative power of expressive art, contributed to the client's ongoing journey of self-reclamation and narrative re-authoring. The client's evolution from internalized shame to a place of empowerment is a testament to an integrative approach's profound impact, especially when tailored to honor the complexity of lived experiences. This case highlights the importance of embracing a multifaceted approach that does not simply aim to reduce symptoms but actively redefines the client's relationship with their body, past, and potential future. By thoughtfully integrating harm reduction, somatic awareness, and expressive art, therapists can help clients rewrite their stories, reclaim their bodies, and ultimately thrive despite the challenges they have faced.

An integrative approach underscores the belief that every client's story is valid and that the journey toward healing can be as creative, fluid, and multifaceted as our identities. The process documented here addresses the immediate need for self-regulation and harm reduction. It sets the stage for ongoing self-care, resilience, and empowerment, transforming lived experiences of marginalization into narratives of hope and strength.[9]

PRACTICE EXAMPLE

Embodied Artmaking

Invite your client to settle into a comfortable, private space with a simple art kit, including paper or canvas, a choice of drawing tools (pencils, charcoal, markers), collage materials (scraps of colored paper, fabric, tape), and paints of varying consistencies.

Begin by guiding them through a few slow, grounding breaths, noticing how the air expands the belly and softens the chest. Then move into a brief, nonjudgmental body scan, naming any areas of tightness, warmth, or emptiness as "here" and "there," without needing to change them.

Without breaking that gentle awareness, invite them to draw a continuous, flowing shape with both hands. Whether spirals, waves, or lines, they let the rhythm of their breath and the feel of the tool in both hands regulate their nervous system as they mirror motions across the page. Next, they choose two or three colors that "feel" like safety, strength, tension, or release and apply them intuitively over or alongside the drawing, perhaps layering watercolor washes to symbolize vulnerability and resilience, or using opaque acrylic strokes to mark boundaries where they wish to feel protected.

As they work, suggest that they pause occasionally to notice any shifts in bodily sensation, such as warmth in their hands, a lightening in their shoulders, or a flutter in their heart, and let that guide their next material choice or brushstroke. If the urge to self-soothe arises, they might gently press a hand to their chest or massage their shoulders, honoring that impulse rather than judging it.

When the image feels "whole enough," invite them to write a single word or short phrase in a corner, something that reminds them of their wisdom or worth ("I am here," "This body knows," "Peace resides within"), and to place it into the composition, acknowledging that harm reduction means any small step toward self-kindness is a victory.

Finally, they sit back, place a hand over their heart, and breathe, with the finished artwork nearby, recognizing that this practice, melding somatic attunement with expressive creation, is something they can return to whenever they need to reconnect mind, body, and creativity in service of their ongoing healing.

5

Liberating Queer Bodies Through Somatic and Expressive Art Therapies

Queer bodies have long been subject to surveillance, regulation, erasure, and violence. Historically, Western medical, mental health, and legal systems have pathologized and policed Queer expressions, rendering societally non-normative bodies and identities as wrong, deviating from the societal norm. The rigid classifications that have emerged from these spaces have not only marginalized Queer individuals but have also sought to discipline their bodies into adhering to predetermined gender and behavioral scripts. Against this backdrop, somatic and expressive arts practices emerge as vital spaces where Queer individuals, through their resilience and strength, can reinhabit their bodies with agency and creativity, challenging dominant narratives and generating new ways of being, feeling, and knowing. These practices forge connections between personal liberation and collective transformation, providing a language that speaks to lived experience.[1] This chapter examines the evolution, theory, and practice behind this therapeutic approach, highlighting its centrality in a cultural moment that values diversity, creativity, and embodied resistance.

Engaging in somatics centers the body's wisdom, engraved in every contour, movement, and breath. It calls for cultivating an acute awareness of sensation, rhythm, and fluidity beneath the surface of everyday interactions with the world. When practiced through a Queer lens, somatics becomes a means of Queering embodiment itself. It refuses the binary logic imposed by heteronormative standards, embraces the fluidity of desire and identity, and honors the full spectrum of bodily experience. Similarly, expressive arts provide venues for the creation of alternative narratives in which Queer lives are rendered not merely legible but celebratory and transformative. In such practices, the body becomes a medium and message, a living archive where cultural memory and political resistance converge.[2]

In recent decades, Queer artists, therapists, and activists have advanced the notion that these embodied practices carry liberatory potential. Reclaiming somatic and artistic expression, rooting them in lived, communal, and creative settings, these therapists reimagine healing not as a return to a stifling status quo but as an unfolding process, dynamic, relational, and fundamentally transformative. Liberation in this framework is not a static endpoint; it is an emergent, continuous process of re-embodiment, a lived reality that is both felt and enacted daily. It is orchestrating a new cultural language of the body, where each gesture can be read as an act of survival and subversion.

The concept of the body as a vibrant, responsive, meaning-making entity resonates deeply with Queer theories that challenge the entrenched dualisms of Western thought, such as mind/body, reason/feeling, and nature/culture, that have historically been used to constrain both identities and expressions.[3] Pioneering feminist theorists have set the stage for rethinking embodiment. Judith Butler's writings on gender performativity, for example, have illuminated how gender identity is continually created through repeated, embodied performances.[4] Susan Bordo's critical work on the body reveals the cultural inscriptions that mark our physical forms.[5] Audre Lorde's famous declaration that "the erotic is power" reconceptualizes bodily pleasure and creative expression as potent forms of resistance. These feminist insights intersect with Queer critiques to propose that the body is an active site of political and social inscription, a canvas on which alternative stories of selfhood and community can be inscribed.[6]

The contributions of other Queer and BIPOC people have further enriched the conversation around somatics. Queer theorists such as Lee Edelman and José Esteban Muñoz have examined how the state and dominant cultural institutions perpetuate disciplinary practices aimed at regulating Queer lives.[7] In parallel, critical interventions in somatic practices, such as the work on somatics by Resmaa Menakem, highlighted how trauma, embodied in the form of chronic stress, pain, or tension, is both a product of and a site for potential liberation.[8] This theoretical framework does not just locate trauma; it envisions the body as a vessel of ancestral memory that can be actively reimagined through creative practice.

For centuries, non-normative modes of being have been systematically erased or devalued through policies and practices that privilege a narrow definition of the "ideal" body. In contrast, somatics and expressive arts create a space where the body's multiplicity is tolerated and celebrated. They challenge the logic of exclusion, inviting a reclamation of bodily autonomy that is inherently political and culturally regenerative. In this view, the body becomes a site where alternative knowledge emerges that negotiates past tensions while mapping out future possibilities.[9] Emphasizing cultural humility and intersectionality, current therapists understand that the body's stories are inseparable from histories of oppression and survival. Cultural humility and intersectionality insist that the processes of embodiment and expression must be approached with sensitivity to the myriad ways in which power operates, whether through racism, sexism, ableism, or heteronormativity. In doing so, these frameworks forge a path toward practices deeply rooted in community histories and experiences, employing somatic inquiry as a method of healing and resistance.[10]

To truly "Queer" somatic and expressive practices is to challenge and destabilize the norms that dictate who is permitted to be visible, safe, or even recognized as having a story worthy of telling. In mainstream wellness culture, dominant narratives often celebrate white, cisgender, able-bodied, and thin embodiments, reproducing a narrow set of ideals that marginalize bodies outside these confines. Queer somatic practices, on the other hand, affirm that lived experience, with all its variability and messiness, is a source of strength and creativity. They celebrate the diversity of Queer bodies, so everyone feels included and valued. Artistic expression within Queer spaces becomes an act of radical reclamation. Whether through dance, sound, or visual media, every act of creative embodiment resists the forces that seek to reduce complex lives into neat, marketable images. In these spaces, movement is a multisensory ritual that speaks to individual experience and collective memory. This aesthetic of resistance celebrates contradiction, ambiguity, and disruption. Rather than conforming to standards of legibility or coherence, Queer expressive practices thrive on the tension between self-definition and fluid identity. Their disruptive energy reclaims power from normalized narratives and opens possibilities for alternative modes of relational existence.[11]

At its core, the act of movement in Queer spaces is political. Every breath taken freely, every spontaneous gesture, and every rhythmic pattern articulated on a stage of collective experience represents a rejection of the disembodied norms that characterize modern society. In a culture that often equates stillness with order and silence with discipline, the spontaneous kinetic expression of Queer bodies becomes a proclamation of freedom. Ranging from the subtle undulations of breathwork to the exuberant outbursts of musical improvisation, this movement challenges the enforcement of rigid structures and affirms the expansive potential of bodily self-determination. We can see this in the work of artists like Keith Haring and the ACT UP movement.[12]

Moreover, these practices emphasize relationality and interconnection. Liberation is not achieved in isolation but is continuously negotiated through embodied interactions among individuals. The presence of another body in movement, the shared space where gestures and expressions collide, forms a collective ecology in which each participant becomes both teacher and student. This mutual witnessing of vulnerability, resilience, and joy creates embodied knowledge that nurtures the spirit of resistance.[13] Within these relational containers, the boundaries between self and others are softened, which allows for a more fluid and dynamic conception of identity and community.

Queer somatic practices also link the present to both ancestral memories and future aspirations. Recalling and reinterpreting historical trauma through movement and creative reenactment transform pain into an archive of potential power. In these practices, the body is read as a site of suffering and a storehouse of wisdom and energy. This living repository remembers the past and channels its insights toward the future. Here, liberation unfolds not as a singular moment of breakthrough but as an ongoing performance, a choreography where each movement is steeped in meaning and charged with the promise of transformation.[14]

The subversive nature of these practices extends into the realm of aesthetics. They reject the sanitized representations imposed by mass media and dominant culture, opting for a rich mixture of images, sounds, and gestures that defy conventional categorization. This aesthetic revolt destabilizes rigid identities and creates a vibrant cultural milieu where difference is celebrated and multiplicity is the norm. The interplay of shadow and light in a dramatic dance sequence, the raw textures of improvised soundscapes, or the bold brushstrokes in a spontaneous mural, each modality speaks to resistance against conformity, proposing alternative narratives that are as diverse as they are powerful.[15]

As somatic and expressive arts expand within therapeutic, educational, and community domains, it is imperative that they resist assimilation into structures that perpetuate normative and exclusionary ideals. Instead of seeking legitimacy solely through conventional clinical models or commercial incentives, these practices should be envisioned as foundational elements in the broader struggle for justice, inclusion, and liberation. They are not peripheral tools or adjunct techniques but core practices that embody alternative ways of understanding and living in the world.

This means a radical change in how we conceive of healing and care for therapists in therapeutic and community settings. Cultivating spaces that actively affirm Queer and trans embodiments involves a commitment to ongoing self-reflection and a willingness to dismantle internalized norms. Therapists must be prepared to navigate the complexities of lived experience, holding space for vulnerability and strength and fostering a climate of inclusivity that honors difference rather than attempting to normalize it. They must take creative risks and reinstate playfulness as a core element of the healing process. By embracing what might appear as disruption or chaos, therapists can catalyze deeper engagement with the embodied self, allowing for an organic unfolding of personal truth.[16]

Ultimately, to center somatic and expressive arts in the context of Queer liberation is to affirm that the body is not simply a biological entity subject to external control but a vibrant, evolving site of possibility. It is a declaration that healing, and by extension, living authentically, is about embracing the full and messy reality of what it means to be human. Through the interplay of movement, breath, sound, and image, we rediscover that our bodies carry marks of past traumas and the seeds of future transformation. They are texts written in flesh, resisting, remembering, and reimagining the world at every turn.

In a world that often demands disembodiment, intellectual detachment, and the suppression of raw, unfiltered life, somatic and expressive arts provide a counter-narrative, a rejuvenation of the self that is as political as it is personal. For Queer communities, these practices are potent rituals of thriving. They are acts of love in motion, declarations of resistance in rhythm, and assertions of freedom in form. In every collective breath, a quiet revolution unfolds in each spontaneous gesture, one that is as ancient as it is urgently modern, as deeply personal as it is widely political.

By embracing the diversity of bodily expression, we affirm that liberation is not a solitary achievement but a shared journey. The language of the body, its movements, sensations, and resonances, speaks to an inherent desire to live freely and authentically. This calls on us to reimagine a world where the body is honored in all its multiplicity, healing is an act of collective reawakening, and every sensory experience is a pathway to transformative change. In the larger picture of cultural production and social justice, somatics and expressive arts practices are luminous beacons of possibility. They offer an expansive, inclusive, and continuously evolving vision of liberation. As we move forward into uncertain futures, these embodied practices can help us navigate the complexities of identity, power, and resistance in a deeply personal and inherently political manner. Thus, by reclaiming the body as a site of wisdom and possibility, Queer somatics and expressive arts remind us that every movement is both an act of defiance and an affirmation of life.

This chapter calls for a radical reimagining of our relationship to the body, so that we can see healing as the creation of ever-unfolding futures. It is an invitation to live in the fullness of our embodied truth, to challenge the constraints imposed upon us, and to participate in a collective liberation that honors the diverse, dynamic, and undeniably powerful nature of the Queer body.

By integrating somatic therapy and expressive artistic practices spanning music, dance and movement, studio art, theater, and photography, Queer individuals have constructed new spaces of healing and transformation. These practices are routes to personal well-being and the building blocks for a broader politics of body liberation.

Historically, Queer people were forced to navigate a society where their bodies were often seen as aberrant and, at times, criminal. In reaction to pervasive stigmatization and marginalization, the Queer community turned to creative expression as a form of resistance. Art became an act of defiance, a way to subvert hostile social norms and reclaim space for authentic self-expression. Early Queer artistic movements, from the underground club scenes of the 1970s to the vibrant street performances and guerrilla theater of later decades, laid the groundwork for the interwoven practices of somatic and expressive art therapies that we recognize today.

Art and activism were intrinsically linked during these formative periods. Queer creatives used every medium available to them, music, dance, performance, and visual arts, to forge communities of mutual support and to articulate a vision of liberation that challenged heteronormative expectations of what a body should be. These historical precedents are essential for understanding today's integrative therapeutic practices; they reveal how the creative impulse has always served to heal personal wounds and as a communal survival and empowerment strategy.

The evolution of somatic and expressive art therapies in the Queer context is deeply rooted in contemporary theoretical perspectives on the body and identity. Judith Butler's seminal work on gender performativity challenges the notion of fixed gender identities and posits that gender is continuously constituted through repeated acts.[17] This paradigm shift suggests that the body is not a static canvas but a dynamic, transformative element in identity construction. Somatic therapies, which emphasize the body's lived experience, dovetail naturally with Butler's ideas, encouraging individuals to understand and reframe their bodily sensations as acts of creation rather than mere reactions to external pressures.

Complementing Butler's insights, theorists like José Esteban Muñoz have introduced the idea of "disidentification" as a method of negotiating cultural norms.[18] According to Muñoz, Queer subjects can engage with and transform dominant cultural symbols, repurposing them to subvert normative discourses. This process is inherently embodied, operating in the physical expression of dance and movement and the visual language of art. The interplay between theoretical approaches and clinical practice is evident in the way somatic therapy enables Queer individuals to locate and process trauma while simultaneously rediscovering the inherent wisdom of their body.[19]

At the heart of somatic and expressive art therapy is the conviction that healing must attend to the body as much as it does to the mind. Whereas traditional therapeutic modalities have privileged cognitive and verbal expression, somatic and expressive approaches recognize the myriad ways in which trauma, stress, and identity are inscribed on the body. In clinical settings, therapists are increasingly trained to view physical sensations, muscle tension, breath rhythms, and energy flows as rich data sources on a patient's emotional state. This embodied awareness is particularly significant in Queer contexts, where historical and ongoing traumas can lead to disconnection from one's physical self. By re-centering the body in therapy, clinicians help individuals experience a fuller range of emotional release and transformation.

Expressive art therapy reinforces this shift by using creative practices as a medium to articulate and transform internal experiences that defy easy description. When words fail to capture the complexity of Queer experiences, art offers an alternative vocabulary, a visual or performative language that speaks directly to the soul. Whether through the improvisational flow of dance, the evocative brushstrokes in a painting, or the dynamic energy of a musical composition, these art forms operate as both diagnostic tools and healing modalities; participants can witness and ultimately transform the legacies of trauma that reside in their bodies.

Somatic therapy recognizes that the body retains memories of experiences, emotions, and traumas that may not be fully accessible through conventional talk therapies. Drawing from disciplines as varied as body psychotherapy, yoga, and mindfulness, it encourages therapists to observe and interpret the signals encoded in their clients' musculature, breath, and bodily movements. In the realm of Queer health, somatic therapy has proven particularly transformative, as it offers clients a way to reconnect with a body that has been a target of external judgment or violence.

By working through physical sensations rather than solely relying on verbal narratives, somatic therapy opens up a space where healing is multilayered. For instance, a simple practice like mindful breathing can be powerfully grounding for an individual who has internalized external hostility. Over time, such interventions help create an embodied experience of safety and acceptance, a counter-narrative to the body shame that many Queer people have experienced. This process alleviates physical tension and facilitates a profound reconnection to self, where the body is recognized as a vessel of both vulnerability and strength.[20]

In somatic practice, physical manifestations, be they tension in the shoulders or a quickened heartbeat, are not symptoms to be suppressed but messages to be heeded. Therapists skilled in somatic approaches teach clients to "listen" to these bodily signals as one might listen to a piece of music, interpreting rhythms and cadences that reveal deeper emotional landscapes. With practice, clients learn that the body, in its myriad responses, holds the keys to unlocking long-buried traumas and reclaiming personal power. For Queer individuals, whose bodies have long been politicized or manipulated by external forces, this embodied listening becomes an act of defiance, a declaration that the self is not defined by external judgment but by its own lived truth. This emphasis on reclaiming personal power can make the audience feel empowered and in control of their healing journey.

Somatic Techniques for Experiential Healing

Mindful movement, breathwork, body scanning, somatic experiencing, and expressive moment practices are all examples of techniques that support the core principles of somatic therapy and offer tangible methods for integrating body-mind awareness.

Drawing on principles from yoga, tai chi, and contemporary dance, conscious movement practices encourage participants to engage with their body in an intentional and exploratory manner. Movements, whether slow and deliberate or spontaneous and free, can help release deeply held tension and promote an embodied sense of freedom.[21]

Controlled breathing exercises serve as gateways to understanding bodily states. By modulating their breath, individuals can alter their emotional states, reduce anxiety, and create a direct pathway from the physical to the emotional. Breathwork is often integrated into sessions to ground participants before delving into more challenging emotional terrain.

In body scan practices, participants are guided through a meditative process of focusing sequentially on different body parts. This systematic approach cultivates awareness of where stress or discomfort is held, allowing the individual to address these sensations with compassion rather than judgment.[22]

Somatic experiencing is a method for gradually releasing trauma stored in the nervous system. By encouraging clients to experience sensations in a controlled and safe environment, this technique helps dissolve the physical residues of traumatic encounters.[23]

All these practices incorporate improvisational fluid movement and encourage the spontaneous expression of internal states. They allow clients to witness their bodies' stories unfold in a choreography of release and renewal. For Queer individuals, these practices provide a counterhegemonic narrative, inviting clients to see their bodies as living art capable of transformation and resistance. Engaging with the body in these mindful and creative ways becomes an empowering ritual that transforms shame into pride and disempowerment into liberation.

Expressive art, whether painting, collage, sculpture, music, or performance, can enhance somatic practices, and it is particularly salient for Queer communities, because language alone may not be able to encompass the complexities of identity, desire, and trauma. Art opens up alternative avenues of communication that are more fluid, spontaneous, and intrinsically linked to the individual's lived experience. Thus, the creative process becomes not simply an act of making something beautiful but a psychological and emotional reclamation.

Music has long been a cornerstone of Queer cultural expression. Its capacity to evoke deep emotional responses and transform personal narratives makes music a powerful tool in expressive art therapy. In therapeutic settings, music is utilized for its aesthetic qualities and as a medium through which suppressed feelings can be voiced. In group or individual sessions, activities may include guided improvisation on instruments, vocal exercises, or songwriting. These practices have the dual effect of validating personal experiences and fostering a shared sense of community. For example, a therapeutic circle involving collective singing or drumming can generate a profound connection among participants, reinforcing that the individual's struggle is part of a larger, communal journey toward healing and celebration. Moreover, creating music challenges mainstream narratives that dictate narrow definitions of beauty and talent. It subverts traditional musical hierarchies by highlighting diversity in sound, rhythm, and lyrical content, the very qualities that make Queer musical expression so vital and revolutionary.[24]

Dance is one of the most immediate ways the body communicates its inner state. For the Queer community, dance has frequently served as an emancipatory practice, a space where gendered and heteronormative constraints can be broken apart and reassembled into forms that celebrate fluidity and diversity. Within the context of expressive art therapy, dance and movement allow participants to bypass the limitations of language and access a more primal, instinctual form of expression. Therapeutic interventions include structured dance routines, free-form improvisation, or group movement exercises that highlight the physicality of emotion. These practices emphasize that every gesture, even as simple as a sway or a gesture of defiance, holds narrative power. Participants learn to view their body as an instrument of expression, capable of conveying complex emotions and stories without uttering a single word. Dance, therefore, becomes a mirror for internal states and a stage for celebrating nonconformity. It underscores a fundamental principle of somatic and art therapies: The body is a living archive of resilience, and its movements are as significant as any spoken language.

Visual art offers a unique modality for self-exploration and expression. In studio art therapy, painting, drawing, and collage allow individuals to externalize complex internal landscapes onto a tangible medium. For Queer individuals, who may experience a disconnect between societal representations of the body and their lived reality, studio art serves as an act of reclaiming personal narrative and identity. Engaging with materials like acrylics, charcoal, or clay, clients are invited to experiment with color, texture, and form to portray their internal experiences. The creation process is inherently iterative; each brushstroke or sculptural form serves as a record and a transformation of past pain into emergent beauty. Through this creative process, participants craft imagery that challenges traditional beauty standards. Studio art therapy thus becomes a deliberate act of resistance, a way to visualize and affirm the diversity, complexity, and worth of Queer embodiment. It invites the artist to occupy their definition of beauty, rewriting narratives that have long excluded the fullness of their being.[25]

Photography is a tool for both documentation and creative expression in the Queer community. In many ways, capturing an image affirms presence: a declaration that one exists and deserves to be seen. Expressive art therapy sessions incorporating photography encourage participants to explore self-portraiture and collaborative projects that present an alternative narrative to mainstream representations. Techniques in therapeutic photography include guided photo walks, the creation of themed visual diaries, or studio sessions designed to experiment with light and shadow. These practices empower individuals to control how they are represented, challenging the historically negative or stereotypical portrayals imposed by external media. By reframing the act of looking, whether at oneself or through the lens, the photographer reclaims the gaze, converting vulnerability into a confident stance of self-affirmation. The images produced in this process are not merely art objects; they are visual testaments to transforming internal landscapes of shame into vibrant declarations of joy, resilience, and empowerment.[26]

Across its many forms, art has always been inherently political, challenging the status quo and questioning established truths. Within Queer contexts, artistic practice becomes a potent act of political resistance, one that works to dismantle the barriers imposed by heteronormative and cis-normative ideologies. Every musical composition, dance performance, work of visual art, theatrical experiment, or photographic project is a direct challenge to the narrow definitions of beauty and legitimacy that dominate mainstream culture. By giving voice to histories of marginalization and by celebrating unconventional bodies, Queer art transforms the act of self-expression into a form of protest. It asserts unequivocally that diverse embodiments, irrespective of age, gender, ability, or appearance, are not only valid but are essential to the richness of human experience. Creating becomes a manifesto: a declaration that everybody has the right to exist, express, and flourish. This politicization of art, far from being a fringe phenomenon, is at the heart of contemporary movements for social justice and cultural transformation.

Collective Practices for Healing

One of the most potent ways to integrate somatic and expressive art therapies in Queer communities is a collective practice. When individuals come together to create art through collaborative theater, dance, or art projects, they forge a shared narrative that transcends the individual. Collective practices serve as a communal archive of resistance; they record the experiences of multiple lives and reinforce the idea that healing is not only a solitary act but also an interdependent process. Group sharing, collaborative creative projects, and peer support circles enhance people's sense of belonging. In such spaces, even the most vulnerable expressions are received as legitimate and powerful forms of communication. The therapeutic process, therefore, becomes a mutually created community where healing is both an individual and collective journey.

In communal workshops, for example, participants might engage in a series of movement explorations that lead to an impromptu performance. The synergy created in such moments amplifies personal healing by transforming it into a communal celebration of diversity and resilience. These shared rituals underscore a fundamental principle: that creation is intrinsically social. In Queer communities, this social dimension provides a counterbalance to isolation and affirms that the liberation of the body is inherently bound up with the liberation of the community. Central to the transformative power of these artistic and therapeutic practices is the reconfiguration of what the body means.

In dominant cultural narratives, the body is too often rendered as a site of imperfection, something to be disciplined, corrected, or hidden. Queer art and somatic therapies, however, reframe the body as a source of intrinsic wisdom and as a repository of lived history. As more therapists embrace integrative and multimodal approaches, new methods that promise even deeper levels of healing and liberation are emerging. Innovations are seen in the refinement of traditional techniques and in developing novel practices that draw on digital technology, interdisciplinary collaboration, and cross-cultural exchange.[27]

Community-led initiatives are pivotal in shaping these emerging practices, in particular. By centering the voices and experiences of Queer people, therapists can create therapeutic and creative spaces that are not only profoundly resonant but also empowering. Community-led projects ensure that the evolution of therapeutic practices remains sensitive to the cultural, social, and political realities of those who have long been marginalized. In doing so, they chart a course toward a future where inclusivity drives healing, and the arts continue to catalyze systemic change.[28]

Integrating social justice into clinical practices is another area ripe for further exploration. At their core, somatic and expressive art therapies are inherently political acts that call to reclaim individual and collective autonomy over the body. Future developments in these fields may increasingly incorporate social justice frameworks to ensure that the therapeutic process remains attentive to personal healing and broader societal change. By aligning clinical practices with community activism, therapists and artists can work together to challenge institutional norms, promote equitable healthcare, and foster cultural environments where every body is celebrated. As practices evolve, the transformative promise of embodied creativity continues to inspire new generations of Queer individuals and allies alike. The notion that every movement, every musical note, every brushstroke, every theatrical performance, and every photograph contributes to the collective reimagining of what it means to be human is at the core of contemporary artistic and therapeutic innovation. Future research and practice in these fields will likely further elucidate how creative expression catalyzes personal and social transformation, a line of inquiry that promises scientific insight and profound cultural impact.[29]

Somatic therapy, expressive art therapy, and body liberation represent a merging of practices that challenge the constraints of traditional healing modalities. Together, these approaches assert that healing must be embodied and creative, intertwining the physical, emotional, and artistic dimensions of human experience. Through the engaging modalities of music, dance and movement, studio art, theater, and photography, Queer communities are actively redefining what it means to heal, to resist, and to exist. Every innovative technique in somatic therapy, from mindful breathing to expressive movement, reminds us that the body is a dynamic source of resilience and creativity. Similarly, the transformative power of expressive art therapy lies in its capacity to articulate what cannot be spoken, a reconfiguration of internal narratives that challenge the societal norms that have long marginalized non-normative bodies (by society's standards).[30]

The ongoing dialogue between individual experience and collective creativity highlights a critical aspect of Queer culture: the conviction that liberation is both a personal journey and a communal project. In embracing practices that foster holistic healing, Queer communities are reclaiming their narratives and also actively challenging mainstream representations of identity, beauty, and worth. Art becomes not just an act of self-expression but an act of survival and revolution, a tangible assertion that every body, in all its diversity and complexity, is a power source. By acknowledging the interconnectedness of body, mind, and art and by committing to practices that celebrate diversity and resist marginalization, we lay the groundwork for a future where healing is a continuous, collaborative process, one that honors the full spectrum of human experience and champions the freedom of everybody to be.[31]

Case Example: Expressive Art Therapy for Queer Body Liberation

This case study delves into the profound and transformative impact of an integrative expressive art therapy approach with Queer body liberation. The client, an Indian American woman in her forties (she/her), presents with complex challenges that stem from internalized body image issues, cultural disconnection, and the struggle to fully embrace her Queer identity within a multifaceted relational context. Despite a successful career in the medical field, she wrestles with feelings of alienation from the Queer culture she admires, an alienation that is compounded by her personal life: She is married to a man while also being involved in a polyamorous relationship with three partners (a cis-woman, a cis-man, and a trans woman).

This case study details the journey of reconnecting with Queer art movements and the power of ballroom culture. The interventions centered on card collage, music, dance, and movement to foster somatic release. They facilitated a deeper integration of her self-image with the liberatory narratives she found inspiring. Throughout therapy, these modalities served as both an expressive outlet and a medium through which the client could reclaim her narrative, ultimately achieving a renewed sense of embodiment and self-acceptance.

The client's cultural heritage is a complex mosaic of traditional South Asian values and contemporary American influences. Growing up within this bicultural framework, she experienced early exposure to South Asian familial expectations and the broader American cultural narrative, which often conflicted with the more fluid, self-determined forms of expression she encountered in Queer spaces.

Professionally, the client has enjoyed a stable career in the medical field, a domain that demands precision, discipline, and adherence to established protocols. While this professional identity is a source of pride, it also contributes to an internalization of perfectionism and a disconnection from more spontaneous, creative aspects of her personality. The rigorous structure of her work life leaves little room for exploring her identity's emotional and artistic dimensions, further isolating her from the creative communities that might otherwise have provided support and inspiration.

Her personal life adds another layer of complexity. In both her marriage and her polyamorous relationship, she navigates an intricate web of relational dynamics. These relationships have provided her with love and support and also posed challenges in integrating different facets of her identity. The societal pressures and cultural expectations, both from her family and within broader societal norms, have often conflicted with her internal vision of Queer liberation and self-expression. The tension between fulfilling social expectations and exploring a liberated Queer identity has been a recurrent theme throughout her life.

A recurring challenge for the client has been a deep-seated struggle with body image. Despite professional success and loving relationships, she has harbored persistent feelings of inadequacy and shame regarding her body. These feelings were exacerbated by a sense of disconnection from the very Queer culture that celebrated difference and defied normative expectations. While she revered the works and legacies of iconic Queer and feminist artists and activists, she also found it difficult to relate their narratives to her own lived experience. The disconnect left her feeling isolated and uncertain about her place within the Queer community.

The client's journey is best understood through intersectionality. Her experience as an Indian American woman, coupled with her nontraditional relationship structure and internalized body image concerns, required a nuanced approach that acknowledged the multiple layers of marginalization and empowerment simultaneously.

This client's intervention was built around four primary creative modalities: collage cards, music, dance/movement, and the integration of Queer art movements. Collage cards are a form of creative expression that uses visual art to externalize inner experiences. The client pieced together images, symbols, and words that represent her internal world, thereby creating a visual narrative that bridges the gap between her internal struggles and the broader cultural narratives she admires. Music has the power to evoke emotional responses, trigger memories, enhance movement, and facilitate somatic experiences. For this client, music selected from Queer and activist traditions provided both comfort and a call to liberation. Movement practices are essential in helping individuals reconnect with their bodies. Dance offers a way to transcend the limitations of verbal expression and access deep-seated emotions. The client's choice to incorporate elements of ballroom culture, which celebrates Queer identity and defies normative expectations, was instrumental in fostering a sense of belonging and liberation. By engaging with Queer artists and activism, the therapy sought to contextualize her personal experience within a broader historical and cultural framework. This integration highlighted the intersections between art, politics, and personal liberation.

These modalities were chosen for their capacity to engage both the body and the mind in the healing process. Especially for clients dealing with body image issues and cultural disconnection, traditional talk therapy alone may be insufficient. Creative therapies offered an alternative by inviting this client to explore her inner life through tangible, sensory experiences. The combined use of card collage, music, and dance allowed her to experience a form of somatic release, where emotions could be expressed nonverbally and experienced in her body. This was critical in transforming her perception of her body from a source of shame to a symbol of resistance and beauty.

The initial stage of therapy focused on building trust and establishing a safe, nonjudgmental space. Given the complexity of the client's identity and experiences, it was important to create an environment where she could express herself freely. Early sessions involved open discussions about her cultural background, relationship dynamics, and the disconnect she felt from the Queer art movements that had long inspired her. During these sessions, I validated her experiences, emphasizing the importance of honoring both her heritage and her Queer identity. A key aspect of this stage was setting intentions for therapy. The client articulated her desire to overcome internalized body shame, reconnect with Queer cultural narratives, explore creative avenues for self-expression, and build a bridge between her identity and the broader liberatory movements in Queer art and activism.

Card collage is an inherently introspective process and invites individuals to engage with their unconscious material. For this client, collage became a metaphor for reconstructing her identity, a method of taking fragmented parts of herself and weaving them into a coherent narrative that celebrated her unique experience. In therapy sessions, materials such as magazines, photographs, scissors, glue, and paper were available for spontaneous creation. Each session began with a guided imagery exercise aimed at centering the client and inviting her to explore her inner landscape. The imagery often drew from elements of nature, urban life, and historical moments from Queer culture. She selected images that resonated with her emotional state, body image, and cultural heritage. As she arranged these elements on stock cards, the process became a dialogue between her conscious self and her repressed emotions. After each collage session, the client and therapist discussed the emerging themes. This debriefing was crucial for linking the visual narratives to her personal history and the broader cultural narratives of Queer resistance and liberation.

Creating card collages enabled the client to externalize her internal struggles and reframe her body image. She began to see her body as a canvas that bore the marks of her experiences, each scar and curve telling a story of survival and defiance. The collages also served as a tangible reminder of her connection to Queer art movements, as recurring symbols from artists like Frida Kahlo and Keith Haring appeared organically in her work. Over time, these visual narratives became a source of empowerment, helping her reclaim her body as a site of beauty and resilience (see Figures 11 and 12).

Music was integrated into the therapeutic process as a stimulus for movement and a means of emotional regulation. The client's playlist was

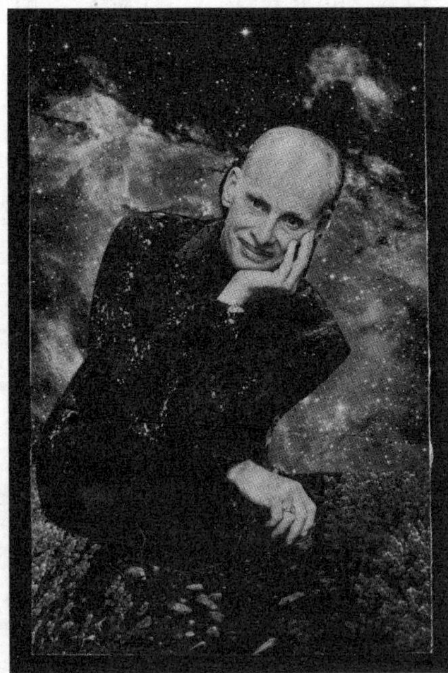

Figure 11. Collage card 1

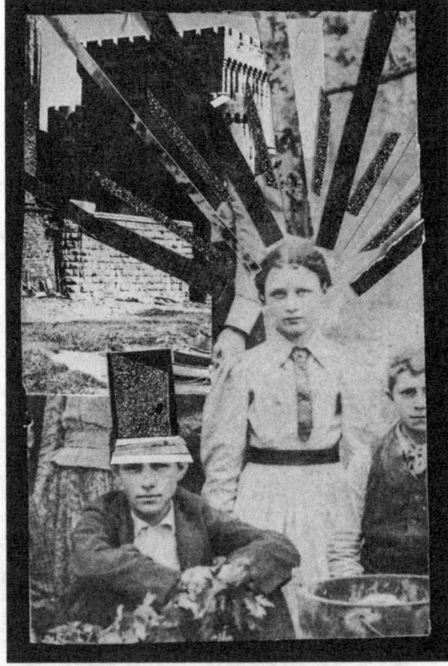

Figure 12. Collage card 2

curated to include tracks that resonated with the themes of Queer liberation, activism, and personal transformation. Music from different eras, ranging from the anthems of ACT UP to the vibrant pop culture influenced by Andy Warhol, provided a rhythmic and emotional underpinning that complemented her creative endeavors. Songs associated with Queer activism and empowerment were introduced early in the process. These tracks served as auditory cues that invoked the historical struggles and triumphs of Queer communities. I worked with the client to create personalized playlists for different stages of therapy, such as introspective card collage sessions or energizing movement practices. By exploring the lyrics, instrumentation, and overall mood of each piece, she learned to attune to her emotional state. Music became a bridge between her internal experiences and the external expressions of joy, sorrow, and liberation.

One of the intervention's most transformative aspects was how dance and movement facilitated somatic release. For this client, movement was not simply a physical activity but a way to reconnect with a part of herself that had been suppressed by years of internalized criticism and societal expectations. In the therapeutic context, the body became a medium for storytelling and self-reclamation.

Particularly significant was the client's choice to integrate elements of ballroom. With its roots in Black and Latino Queer communities, ballroom is renowned for its celebration of difference, creativity, and defiance against mainstream beauty standards. This style's dynamic, expressive movements resonated with her need to break free from the confines of conventional body image norms. Sessions began with simple warm-up exercises, gradually becoming more expressive, free-form movements. I encouraged her to experiment with different dance forms, drawing on the fluidity and dramatism of ballroom routines. The client also learned to tune in to her bodily sensations and emotions through guided movement sessions. Techniques such as body scanning and mindful movement helped her identify areas of tension and emotional blockages. The dance sessions culminated in periods of uninhibited expression, where she was free to move as she wished, guided by the music and her internal impulses. These moments of release were pivotal in dismantling long-held narratives of body shame, replacing them with experiences of joy, power, and liberation.

Throughout several sessions, the client reported a marked improvement in her body awareness and self-perception. The act of dancing, particularly in a style that celebrated Queer identity, allowed her to reclaim her body in a way that was both physical and symbolic. The movement provided a channel for emotional catharsis and a daily reminder that her body was a site of resilience, capable of transformation through expressive, liberatory practices.

An essential component of the intervention was connecting the client's journey with the broader historical context of Queer art and activism. By integrating discussions and visual explorations of key artworks and cultural moments, the client could situate her own experience within a larger context of resistance, beauty, and creativity. These therapeutic sessions included reflective discussions on the works of Keith Haring, Jean-Michel Basquiat, Frida Kahlo, and Andy Warhol. We examined each artist's work for both its aesthetic qualities and its political and cultural significance. I encouraged her to reflect on how these artists had challenged societal norms and redefined beauty, identity, and resistance. She engaged in visual analysis exercises using reproductions of iconic works. She identified recurring themes, vibrancy, defiance, and vulnerability, and discussed how these themes resonated with her struggles and triumphs. The sessions highlighted parallels between the historical context of Queer activism (exemplified by ACT UP) and the client's present-day experience. This linkage helped her see that her journey was part of a continuum of resistance, a personal story embedded within a broader cultural narrative of Queer liberation.

By drawing connections between her life and the legacies of these influential figures, she began to view her body as a repository of history, power, and potential. The artistic and activist narratives counterbalanced the internalized criticisms she had long carried, reinforcing a new self-image rooted in strength and beauty. This case underscores the transformative power of creative therapies. Card collage, music, dance, and movement served as modalities for emotional release and as instruments for self-exploration and redefinition. The creative process allowed the client to externalize her inner conflicts, transforming abstract feelings of shame and disconnection into concrete, visual, and physical expressions. Through art and movement, she could rewrite her narrative and reclaim the liberatory power inherent in her body.

While the intervention was ultimately successful, several challenges emerged along the way. The client's deep-seated cultural beliefs regarding body image and propriety were not easily dismantled. Many early sessions required us to carefully navigate internalized values reinforced over decades. The therapeutic process had to balance respect for her cultural heritage with the need to challenge and expand limiting beliefs. Initially, the client felt uncomfortable using her body as an expression site. Years of conforming to professional norms and societal expectations had left her habitually suppressing bodily movement. Over time, however, gradual exposure and the safe context of therapy helped her overcome her resistance. The client's multifaceted identity, balancing traditional cultural norms, professional expectations, and a liberated Queer identity, required an approach that could honor each dimension. This complexity demanded continuous dialogue and reflective practice in therapy and her personal life.

Several factors contributed to the overall success of this creative and embodied intervention. By addressing both the mind and the body, it allowed for a comprehensive exploration of identity and self-worth. The synergy between creative expression and somatic awareness helped the client change her relationship with her body. Grounding the therapy in the rich traditions of Queer art and activism provided a broader context for healing. The client's ability to see herself in the lineage of celebrated figures and movements was a potent reminder of her strength and resilience. The flexibility to adapt interventions, ranging from visual art to movement-based therapies, ensured the client could engage with the process authentically and resonantly. This personalized approach was key in overcoming early resistance and facilitating deeper emotional work.

This case supports the notion that the body is an active participant in the cognitive and emotional processes of healing. The client's transformation through movement underscores the validity of somatic therapies in addressing psychological issues. Card collage and other creative modalities function as tools for narrative reconstruction. By reassembling the fragments of her identity, the client created a new, empowering story that integrated her cultural, relational, and personal experiences. The case illustrates the importance of an intersectional approach in therapy. Recognizing and honoring the multiple dimensions of the client's identity allowed for a more nuanced and effective intervention that respected her entire lived experience.

Throughout therapy, the client reported significant improvements in her perception of her body. Engaging in collage allowed her to view her physical form as a dynamic and resilient canvas that bore the marks of her life's journey rather than symbols of failure or shame. The integration of movement and dance further reinforced these changes, as she experienced firsthand the liberatory effects of reclaiming her bodily expression. One of the most profound outcomes was the client's renewed connection with Queer culture. By integrating historical narratives from ACT UP and the artistic legacies of renowned Queer icons, she began to see her struggles in a larger, more affirming context. This reconnection fostered a sense of belonging and empowerment, mitigating the feelings of isolation that had once plagued her.

The multimodal approach improved her body image and facilitated a broader capacity for emotional expression. Music and movement provided alternative pathways for accessing and processing emotions that had long remained repressed. The client's ability to express herself, both verbally and nonverbally, grew significantly, leading to deeper insights into her internal world and a more integrated sense of self. The therapeutic journey allowed the client to reconcile the various facets of her identity. Rather than compartmentalizing her cultural heritage, professional identity, and Queer self, she learned to integrate these dimensions into a cohesive narrative. This holistic self-understanding became a cornerstone for her journey toward self-acceptance and liberation.

The positive outcomes in this case suggest that ongoing engagement with creative modalities could further consolidate the client's progress. Participating in card collage sessions or art workshops can give her ongoing opportunities for self-expression and reflection. Enrolling in community dance classes, particularly those that celebrate Queer culture such as ballroom sessions, may offer continued somatic release and community support. Ongoing expressive therapy incorporating music could help maintain her emotional balance and further explore the therapeutic potential of sound and rhythm. Given the client's renewed connection with Queer cultural narratives, efforts to build stronger community ties are paramount. The client's continued engagement with local or online Queer art communities can provide a supportive network that reinforces her sense of belonging. Getting involved in Queer activism or volunteer work with organizations that support body positivity can further enhance her connection to the cultural movements that inspire her. Joining support groups that address body image issues and Queer identity can offer additional spaces for sharing experiences and learning from others. She continued mindfulness meditation to help sustain the somatic awareness developed through dance and movement, reinforcing the mind-body connection. She also began incorporating yoga or other forms of somatic therapy into her life separate from sessions because they deepen her ability to listen to her body, manage stress, and maintain a positive self-image. The client was encouraged to keep a reflective journal documenting her ongoing experiences, creative outputs, and emotional insights. Journaling can serve as a personal archive of her journey and a tool for continuing self-assessment, ensuring that therapeutic gains are sustained over time.

The client's journey illustrates how creative therapies can address deeply rooted issues of body image and cultural disconnection. By harnessing the expressive power of art and movement, the therapeutic intervention enabled her not only to overcome long-held negative beliefs but also to celebrate her identity within a broader context of Queer resistance and liberation. As the mental health field continues to evolve, integrating creative and embodied practices into therapeutic models holds promise for enriching the lives of individuals navigating complex intersections of identity.

Reimagining Healing Through Queer Embodied Liberation

At the heart of Queer body liberation is healing trauma. Trauma does not happen in a vacuum. It is both an individual and a collective experience where bodies exist in ways that accumulate trauma over time. Part of that healing is creating brave spaces where we disconnect from the idea of safety when the world is not inherently safe. Another part is adapting and understanding trauma frameworks like healing-centered engagement and using them to create queer sanctuary where expressive arts and somatic therapy support healing from trauma.[32]

Queer individuals, whose bodies are sites of vibrant creativity, community solidarity, and deep vulnerability, demonstrate remarkable courage and resilience.[33] From the exhilaration of first articulations of desire to the deep bonds forged in chosen families, Queer lives are suffused with moments of affirmation and collective resilience. These same bodies are also subjected to both overt and insidious forms of trauma, ranging from hate- and gender-based violence, forced outing, and conversion practices, to chronic experiences of microaggressions, familial rejection, and institutional erasure.[34] Such trauma does not merely reside in memory; it lives on in the nervous system, shaping interoceptive awareness and becoming inscribed in muscular tension, posture, and movement patterns.[35]

Intersectionality further complicates this picture. A Black trans woman's trauma may be compounded by racism and poverty; a queer immigrant may carry intergenerational wounds of displacement alongside anti-Queer stigmatization. Disability status, neurodivergence, and immigration precarity all intersect with hetero- and cis-normative violence to produce embodied stressors that resist singular, one-size-fits-all interventions. Conventional clinical models, often rooted in biomedical paradigms, may inadvertently pathologize the very identities and bodies they aim to heal, reducing rich lived experiences to diagnostic checklists and neglecting the social and cultural resources that sustain Queer communities.[36]

In response, Queer body liberation reframes trauma healing as a process larger than symptom alleviation; it is a radical reclamation of bodily autonomy, pleasure, and collective belonging. Drawing on Queer theory's provocations against fixed identity categories and Black feminism's insistence on the erotic as a source of power, this paradigm insists that healing begins with honoring the body's inherent wisdom and its capacity for creative self-fashioning.[37] Liberation becomes both a means and an end: When Queer bodies are free to move, express, and congregate on their terms, they reclaim agency from structures that have historically sought to regulate and erase them.

To execute this vision in therapeutic and community contexts, Queer body liberation centers three interlocking paradigms. A "brave space" acknowledges that conversations about power, identity, and trauma inevitably evoke discomfort.[38] By co-creating explicit agreements around consent, language, and accountability, brave space transforms potential re-traumatization into collectively held opportunities for growth and solidarity. "Healing-centered engagement" shifts the therapeutic lens from a deficit-focused *What is wrong with you?* to a strengths-based *What has happened to you, and how can your cultural and communal resources guide your healing?*[39] Healing-centered engagement integrates cultural rituals, storytelling, and collective action, positioning Queerness itself and the rich traditions of Queer resistance as primary vectors of resilience. "Queer sanctuary" reimagines both physical and relational environments as intentional hearths of radical hospitality.[40] Sanctuary spaces are designed and held to honor bodily sovereignty, represent diverse queer identities in every sensory dimension, and embed trauma-informed policies that consistently affirm rather than undermine participants' safety.

Queer body liberation departs from traditional trauma models in three fundamental ways.[41] First, it situates healing within embodied and creative practices, recognizing that expressive arts and somatic therapies access dimensions of experience that verbal discourse alone cannot reach.[42] Second, it foregrounds collective and cultural dimensions of resilience, drawing on ballroom culture and drag performance as living archives of embodied resistance.[43] The emphasis on collective and cultural resilience fosters a sense of connection and support among the participants.[44] Third, it adopts an explicitly anti-oppressive and intersectional stance, insisting that attention to race, class, disability, and immigration status is not optional but integral to any genuine therapeutic work with Queer bodies.[45]

Therapeutic Pathways to Queer Body Liberation

Queer liberation is inextricably linked with trauma healing, especially when approached through the body. Trauma, whether acute incidents of anti-Queer violence or the chronic strain of living under heteronormative and cis-normative oppression, deeply impacts the body-mind system. It leaves imprints in the memory, nervous system, muscles, and breath. Survivors often carry trauma in their posture and patterns of tension; as van der Kolk observes, traumatic experiences live on in the body's physiology, beyond conscious recall.[46] For Queer individuals, these burdens are intersectional. The trauma of a white genderqueer person assigned female at birth will differ from that of a Black trans woman or a disabled Queer refugee; each embodies a unique constellation of marginalization and resilience. A Queer trauma-informed approach must therefore attend to the full context of identity, race, class, gender, sexuality, ability, and immigration status, recognizing how multiple oppressions compound to shape the trauma experience.

Somatic and expressive arts therapies directly engage the embodied nature of trauma. Talk therapy alone often cannot reach the wordless terror or dissociation lodged in a survivor's body. Somatic therapies work with bodily sensation, movement, and breath to safely process trauma that is "stuck" in the nervous system.[47] Similarly, expressive arts modalities, such as visual art, movement, dance, drama, music, and poetry, enable clients to externalize and transform pain through the use of metaphor, imagery, and rhythm.[48] A gesture, a brushstroke, or a verse of poetry can give form to experiences that words fail to capture; each creative act becomes a step toward reclaiming the narrative of one's body. For example, a survivor of hate-based violence might literally shake off fear through vigorous dance or sketch the contours of their tension and then reimagine them in color and light. In doing so, their body is no longer merely a site of injury; it becomes a medium of meaning-making and a canvas of empowerment. Research on trauma confirms that engaging the body in therapy (through breath-work, rhythmic movement, etc.) calms dysregulated stress responses and fosters integration between body and mind. In practice, this means that a Queer client might find a grounding ritual, such as a mindful body scan at the start of each session, to help reestablish a sense of safety and control in their skin. Over time, embodied rituals counteract the physiological imprint of trauma, allowing the client to reclaim their body as a sanctuary rather than a battleground.

Critically, healing in this context is not just individual but collective. Queer communities have long cultivated creative and embodied practices as tools of survival and resistance: the cathartic pageantry of the ballroom scene, the protest art of ACT UP, the sacred dances of Two-Spirit traditions, and playful subversion are embodied resistance.[49] These communal practices carry cultural memory and resilience, dances, rituals, and artworks that celebrate Queer existence in defiance of a hostile world.[50] A trauma-informed liberatory approach deliberately taps into these wellsprings of strength. Therapists might encourage clients to draw on their cultural and communal resources: for instance, incorporating voguing movements from ballroom culture into a movement therapy group to channel pride and fierceness. By situating personal healing within a lineage of collective struggle, clients can feel held by something larger than themselves. Their narrative shifts from *I am broken by what happened to me* to *We have survived, and I carry forward our legacy of resilience.* This emphasis on collective context counters the isolation that trauma and minority stress impose. It affirms that healing, like trauma, is a shared experience, one that can be nurtured in brave spaces, healing-centered engagements, and Queer sanctuaries created in collaboration with others. To realize this vision in clinical and community settings, our framework centers these three interlocking paradigms. Each one complements the somatic and expressive modalities by shaping a supportive context for trauma healing and body liberation.

Brave space, initially developed in the context of social justice education, challenges the notion of therapy as a completely "safe" zone and instead emphasizes courageous engagement.[51] In trauma work, especially with Queer clients, there is no guarantee that discussions of identity, power, and hurt will be comfortable; deep healing often stirs discomfort. A brave space acknowledges this reality. Therapists and participants co-create explicit agreements around consent, language, and accountability. For example, a group might agree that if triggering content arises, they will pause, take a breath, and acknowledge it rather than dismiss it. This transforms moments of potential re-traumatization into shared opportunities for growth and healing. In practice, a brave space approach might involve somatic check-ins (*Where are you feeling tension in your body as we begin?*) and embodied grounding exercises used whenever someone feels unsafe. It also entails real-time repair: If a hurtful comment or misgendering occurs, the facilitator encourages acknowledging the impact and processing it (even with a simple ritual, such as placing a hand on one's heart and breathing together). Such practices model that while absolute safety cannot be guaranteed, collective care and accountability will guide the therapeutic space. In a brave space, queer survivors learn that they can voice pain and truth without being ostracized; their vulnerability is met with validation and courageous witnessing rather than silence. This paradigm thus directly addresses trauma's relational wounds: Where trauma once taught the body to cringe or stay silent, the brave space invites it to stand tall and speak, supported by others committed to working through discomfort together.

Healing-centered engagement expands on trauma-informed care by shifting from a pathology lens (*What is wrong with you?*) to a holistic lens: *What happened to you, and what strengths can help you heal?*[52] A strengths-based paradigm is essential for Queer trauma work because it normalizes survivors' responses as adaptive and emphasizes their cultural and community assets in recovery. A healing-centered engagement approach asks, for example, how a Queer client's hypervigilance or distrust has helped them survive in a hostile environment, and how healing can build on the client's existing resilience. In practice, this might mean integrating storytelling, ritual, and collective action into therapy. A clinician might invite a client to create a personal mythology through collage or creative writing, situating their struggles in a hero's journey narrative that highlights courage and hope.

Group programs may include community-building exercises, such as crafting a shared quilt or playlist of empowering songs by Queer artists, thereby leveraging communal creativity as a healing tool. Healing-centered engagement also urges practitioners to leverage cultural rituals relevant to the client: For some, this could be a Pride march turned somatic ritual (marching in place in the therapy office to reclaim the feeling of protest), for others, a spiritual practice like lighting candles for lost Queer lives to process collective grief. By honoring these cultural, spiritual, and environmental contexts of healing, healing-centered engagement posits that trauma cannot be healed in isolation from the broader forces affecting the client's life. Ginwright notes that when community and creativity are foregrounded, trauma is reframed not as an individual pathology but as an injury of oppression that can be healed through collective care and action.[53] In essence, healing-centered engagement treats Queer healing as a communal "living tapestry," continually co-authored by facilitators and participants, woven with expressive arts and body-focused practices that celebrate each person's strengths. This approach not only alleviates distress but actively cultivates joy, agency, and connection as measures of progress. A client's breakthroughs may be marked by moments when they reclaim a sense of bodily safety, such as the first time they dance without fear or the moment they feel pride in stating their pronouns out loud. Healing-centered engagement ensures these victories are recognized and celebrated as fundamental to healing, not incidental. By asking *What does healing look like for you in your culture and community?* it recenters the client as the expert of their own experience and honors Queer wisdom traditions as equal to clinical knowledge.

The concept of Queer sanctuary reimagines the therapeutic milieu itself as a radical safe haven. It extends the idea of "safe space" by infusing it with active affirmation and hospitality for Queer bodies recovering from trauma.[54] In a Queer sanctuary, every aspect of the environment and relationship is intentional.[55] Physically, this could mean therapy spaces adorned with visible Queer symbols and art, diverse books and imagery that reflect all genders and bodies, and a layout that allows clients autonomy over their comfort, with options to sit, stand, move around, or snuggle under a weighted blanket without judgment. Relationally, Queer sanctuary means the facilitator embodies an ethos of radical welcome, greeting each client's whole self with respect and warmth, using correct pronouns and names unwaveringly, and validating identities and experiences that mainstream settings might marginalize. Policies are trauma-informed by design. For instance, there may be clear guidelines against nonconsensual touch, flexible lighting for those with sensory sensitivities, and confidentiality practices especially attuned to the risks that Queer clients face (e.g., extra care with privacy for clients who are not out publicly). Importantly, Queer sanctuary also invokes community care. It encourages building networks of support around the individual: Therapists might coordinate with Queer-competent medical providers, assist in connecting clients to peer support or local Queer groups, and even incorporate trusted loved ones into sessions when appropriate.

The goal is to surround the client with an ecosystem of safety and affirmation so robust that it counteracts the hostile world outside. In such a sanctuary, a Queer trauma survivor can gradually let down their guard, unlearning the expectation of harm that society has taught their body. As they see their bodily sovereignty consistently honored in therapy (for example, the therapist always asking permission before touching in somatic work, or allowing the client to decorate the space with their art), the client's nervous system learns that here *"my body is respected, my identity is celebrated, and I am protected."* Over time, this experience can be internalized, which reduces hypervigilance and enables deeper therapeutic work. Queer sanctuary is thus both a literal space and a metaphorical one: It is the creation of a container where liberation is practiced in the here and now. Every sensory detail and interaction is aligned with the message that Queer lives are sacred, worthy, and safe to inhabit fully. This stands in stark contrast to the outside environments where trauma originated. By consistently affirming safety and dignity, the sanctuary allows trauma to be processed without re-traumatization, laying the groundwork for authentic re-embodiment.

These three paradigms, brave space, healing-centered engagement, and Queer sanctuary, form a triadic framework that connects trauma-informed practice with Queer-affirming liberation. Together, they depart from traditional trauma treatment in several fundamental ways. First, they insist that healing be grounded in embodied and creative practices, rather than being exclusively rooted in verbal or cognitive approaches. Somatic and arts-based therapies access preverbal trauma memories and offer novel avenues for expression, allowing Queer clients to engage with their pain and resilience holistically.[56]

Second, this approach foregrounds the collective and cultural dimensions of healing.[57] It leverages community rituals, shared stories, and creative cultural expressions, including drag and ballroom performance, Queer street art, and music, as integral components of the therapeutic process.[58] A communal focus counters the alienation of trauma and inspires a sense of belonging and support.

Third, a liberation-focused approach maintains an explicitly anti-oppressive, intersectional stance at all times. Rather than treating race, class, disability, or any other identity factor as an afterthought, it integrates these realities into the core of assessment and intervention.[59] Therapists are called to acknowledge power dynamics and systemic injustices openly in session, naming, for example, how racism or transphobia compound a client's trauma, and to validate the client's lived reality. This empowers clients to see their reactions not as personal failures but as understandable responses to unjust conditions.

In sum, the somatic and expressive arts approach to Queer trauma challenges the client and therapist alike to reimagine healing as an act of social justice. By moving, creating, and feeling in brave space, within a healing-centered process, inside a Queer sanctuary, Queer individuals can do more than reduce the pain of what happened to them. They can reclaim their bodies and experiences as sources of strength, rewrite their stories on their terms, and engage in what Lorde famously called the transformation of silence into language and action.[60] In this way, Queer body liberation is not a distant ideal but a lived, embodied reality that emerges through therapy. Trauma is healed by fully inhabiting the body, by harnessing its capacity for creativity, sensation, and connection to pave the way toward personal and collective liberation.

Taken together, healing-centered engagement, brave space, and Queer sanctuary offer more than just complementary frameworks; they create a coherent, forward-looking ecosystem for trauma healing in Queer bodies. When cultural lineage, relational accountability, and sensory safety are intentionally woven together, trauma work becomes a space of affirmation rather than erasure, fostering collective resilience rather than individual burden. Within this integrated container, Queer participants are encouraged to connect with histories of resistance, embrace vulnerability through shared agreements, and inhabit environments that honor the full complexity of their bodies and identities. The expressive arts and somatic therapies enhance this ecosystem, enabling participants to access subconscious layers of experience, reframe embodied narratives, and regulate their nervous system in culturally meaningful ways. Creative processes and rhythmic somatic practices do more than promote expression; they activate agency, coherence, and joy. Through an intersection of cultural, relational, and embodied approaches, trauma healing transforms into a community-centered venture: one that reclaims Queer bodies as spaces of creativity, connection, and liberated becoming.

PRACTICE EXAMPLE

Embodied Drawing and Movement

In a welcoming, nonjudgmental space, invite your client to begin by closing their eyes for a moment and taking three slow, diaphragmatic breaths, noticing how their belly rises and falls and where in their body they feel warmth, tension, tingling, or stillness. Then, without breaking that gentle awareness, have them open their eyes and choose two or three contrasting art materials, perhaps a smooth pastel crayon and a textured collage paper or a fluid watercolor wash alongside a charcoal stick, and use both hands simultaneously to make mirrored or complementary marks across a single page or canvas, allowing the rhythm of their breath to guide the pressure and speed of each stroke.

As color and texture emerge, encourage the client to intermittently pause, place a hand on their chest or belly, and name silently or aloud any sensations that arise ("I feel grounding here," "I notice fluttering there") before returning to the page, letting those felt cues inform their next choice of hue or tear of paper. After a few minutes of this embodied drawing-collage, play a piece of lyric-free music that resonates with the client's desired emotional tone (calming, energizing, or somewhere in between), and invite them to shift into mindful movement: swaying, tracing large arm circles, or stepping side to side in sync with the beat, using the momentum to transform any areas of held tension into fluid release.

Finally, when the artwork feels "complete enough," ask the client to select a single word or short phrase that they notice emerging from both the art and their body ("I am safe," "My body knows," "I claim joy"), write it directly onto the piece, and close by resting a hand over their heart in gratitude for the wisdom of their body and the creative process they have just shared: an integrated somatic and expressive art practice that any person, regardless of background or identity, can return to whenever they need to bridge mind, body, and imagination in support of healing.

6

Queer Bodies, Somatic Practices, and Expressive Arts in Community and Culture

We gather the threads of our exploration to envision what it truly means when a narrative is liberated. Throughout the previous chapters, we have examined how Queer body narratives are shaped by trauma, culture, and personal experience and how somatic and expressive arts therapies can facilitate healing. Now we turn to the culmination of this journey: the liberatory practices that empower Queer individuals and communities to reclaim and rewrite their body stories. Liberating the narrative is not a singular event but an ongoing process of transformation, a dynamic interplay between personal healing and collective change. Here, we delve into five key dimensions of narrative liberation: the use of embodied rituals for Queer healing, the intersectional understanding of Queer identity, the power of community and collective storytelling, the practice of narrative re-authoring as a path to freedom, and the role of expressive art therapies in unshackling Queer body narratives.

Embodied Rituals and the Restoration of Order After Trauma

Healing often requires a return to structure and meaning in the aftermath of chaos. In therapeutic contexts, embodied rituals provide a consistent, grounding framework that allows trauma survivors to process and transform their experiences. Rituals are repeated, intentional actions laden with symbolic significance, from lighting a candle at the start of a session to complex sequences of movement or art-making practiced regularly. These acts help create an "as-if" space where new meanings can be crafted safely. By engaging the body in patterned, mindful activity, rituals offer a container for emotions that might otherwise feel overwhelming and chaotic. The repetition inherent in ritual provides a sense of order for lives that have felt fragmented, and many cultural traditions recognize ritual as a pathway to healing, often symbolizing rebirth, transition, or connection to something greater. In the context of Queer healing, such rituals can be profoundly validating, as they counteract societal messages of shame with experiences of sacredness and self-affirmation.

For Queer individuals who have endured trauma, whether from personal violations or the insidious stress of living in a stigmatizing society, engaging in ritualistic processes can be especially transformative. Consider the grounding practice of breathwork as an example: Rhythmic breathing exercises calm the nervous system, and when done regularly in a therapeutic ritual, they anchor the individual in the present moment and reinforce a safety narrative. Research supports that breath-centered practices can reduce anxiety and support trauma processing by activating the parasympathetic response and fostering mind-body integration.[1] Likewise, mindfulness rituals such as a body scan meditation at the start of each session create a predictable rhythm that soothes the body's alarm systems and signals that one has entered a sanctuary for healing.[2] Over time, these attunement rituals allow clients to reclaim their body as a site of calm and control rather than chaos and fear.

Creative expression can itself become a ritual. The methodical layering of paint on a canvas or the routine of keeping a daily reflective journal serves as self-expression and a stabilizing ceremony of introspection. Repetitive art-making or movement rituals engage sensory memory in a way that verbal discussion alone cannot. Each stroke of color or repeated dance gesture can symbolically represent an element of one's story, pain, resilience, longing, being acknowledged, and being released. For example, the El Duende one-canvas art method invites a client to return to a single canvas over multiple sessions, layering new imagery over old in a ritual of iterative transformation.[3] Through such creative rituals, Queer individuals can externalize and gradually alter internal narratives about their bodies and identities. The careful attention to bodily sensations during these activities, noticing the tension ease in one's shoulders with each brushstroke or the vibrancy of breath during a movement sequence, helps connect conscious intention with unconscious memory. In this way, ritualized creativity fosters a dialogue between the body and the narrative mind, opening a path for new stories of strength to emerge.

It is important to note that rituals in therapy are not about rigidly following rote procedures; instead, rituals are collaboratively shaped with the client to ensure cultural relevance and personal meaning. For Queer clients, this often means drawing on symbols and practices that resonate with their lived experience. A grounding ritual might involve holding an object that affirms their identity while breathing slowly, integrating an external symbol of Queer pride into the embodied practice of self-calming. Such an approach aligns with harm reduction principles in therapy, meeting clients where they are and tailoring practices to what feels affirming and safe. Instead of following a generic relaxation technique, the therapist and client co-create rituals that honor the client's pace and context. A client-led approach ensures that the ritual does not inadvertently replicate the power dynamics of oppression but rather subverts them: The client, often for the first time, becomes the author of their healing ceremony. When a Queer trauma survivor can say, "This calming ritual is mine; it speaks to my story and my body," that is an act of narrative reclamation in and of itself.[4]

The ritual also underscores that healing is a nonlinear, cyclical journey. In many Indigenous and non-Western frameworks, growth is understood as spiraliform; we revisit old wounds at new depths of understanding.

Modern trauma therapy agrees that progress can loop through stages of re-experiencing, releasing, and reframing. By integrating ritual, therapy honors this cyclical nature. A client might return to a grounding mantra or a movement sequence at each new wave of recovery, each time finding new layers of meaning. What begins as a ritual for mere survival can evolve into a ritual of thriving. For example, one person may start a daily practice of journaling about bodily sensations to cope with dysphoria or anxiety; as their narrative liberates, this same ritual may transform into a celebratory space where they record moments of empowerment and body pride. The ritual remains constant, but its significance shifts from coping to celebrating, mirroring the person's transformation.

It is also worth noting that Queer communities have spontaneously developed their healing rituals outside formal therapy. Events like Pride, while celebratory, function for many as annual rituals of affirmation, when the collective act of marching, dancing, and displaying rainbow symbols reinforces a narrative of visibility and joy. On a more intimate scale, there are rituals such as gender transition ceremonies, where friends might gather to witness a transgender person symbolically shed their old name and embrace their new one, perhaps by writing the old name on paper and burning it or cutting a cake decorated with their new name. Though outside the therapy room, these community and personal rituals inform therapeutic practice: A therapist can help a client prepare for or process such events, knitting them into the client's evolving narrative. By recognizing and incorporating the rituals clients already use or cherish in their lives, therapists amplify the resonance of those practices. The message becomes that healing and liberation are not confined to therapy sessions; they permeate everyday life through meaningful actions and traditions.

Embodied rituals thus become tools of transformation. They operate on multiple levels: physiologically regulating the body, psychologically providing comfort through familiarity, and symbolically marking the passage from one narrative state to another. In Queer healing, rituals carry the added weight of subverting oppressive scripts. Each ritualized act of self-care or self-expression, whether a weekly circle dance with Queer peers, a morning affirmation spoken to one's reflection, or a candle lit to honor transgender remembrance, is a statement that the Queer body-mind is worthy of reverence and care. Rituals reintroduce a sense of the sacred into a story that might have been desecrated by prejudice and trauma. Therapists help clients rebuild trust in their bodies by making space for the holy and the intentional. Over time, these practices can yield profound shifts: Nightmares give way to restorative sleep, hypervigilance softens into presence, and numbness melts into a felt sense of vitality. In each shift lies a narrative pivot; the body gradually moves from being a repository of terror to a source of strength and continuity. As Tilsen notes, liberation is not a one-time "breakthrough" but an unfolding process, a choreography where each movement in the healing journey is imbued with significance and the promise of further transformation.[5]

Intersectional Identities in Queer Healing

Queer identity never exists in a vacuum; it continuously intersects with other facets of a person's social location, including race, ethnicity, gender, class, disability, and more. Intersectionality is the analytical framework introduced by Kimberlé Crenshaw that recognizes how overlapping identities produce unique experiences of oppression and resilience.[6] For Queer individuals, an intersectional lens reveals that their narrative of self is shaped not only by homophobia or transphobia but also by the myriad other power dynamics they navigate. A Queer Black transfeminine person, for instance, carries a body narrative woven from threads of racism, sexism, transphobia, and perhaps the ancestral traumas of enslavement or colonization. These elements complicate both the harm experienced and the healing pathways available. In the context of narrative liberation, intersectionality ensures that we do not oversimplify a client's story. Instead, we honor the full complexity of their lived experience, validating that a sense of alienation might stem not just from Queerness but from being

Queer and a person of color and living with a disability, for example. By naming these converging forces, therapists and clients can better locate the sources of trauma.

For example, Queer and transgender people with disabilities often face not only homophobia and transphobia but ableism as well; their stories may include being desexualized by society or struggling for bodily autonomy in medical settings that overlook their identities. Likewise, Indigenous Queer narratives (such as those of Two-Spirit individuals in Native communities) remind us that intersectionality also means navigating the legacy of colonialism and cultural revitalization. These individuals may draw strength from non-Western traditions that historically held sacred roles for gender-nonconforming people, even as they fight contemporary bigotry.

Intersectional awareness is crucial in developing liberatory narratives because it highlights how social injustices contribute to personal trauma. For instance, research on collective trauma in Queer communities notes that while Queer people share some common historical traumas, such as the AIDS crisis or the criminalization of homosexuality, these experiences are further inflected by race, nationality, and class.[7] A gay white man and a gay man of color will both carry the painful narrative of the AIDS epidemic's toll. Still, the latter may also carry intergenerational wounds of racism and medical neglect that compound his experience. Indeed, historical traumas can be passed down in the psyches and bodies of marginalized people, even without direct parent-to-child transmission. Because Queer identity is not usually transmitted through family lineage in the way ethnicity or religion might be, community and cultural channels become the vectors for intergenerational Queer trauma. Stories of past persecution, from the banishment of gender-variant people in history to modern hate violence, form a kind of cultural memory that Queer individuals inherit as part of their identity.[8] These historical narratives can intensify vigilance and shape what feels "allowed" or safe in the present. This may manifest as an ambient sense of caution, shame, or grief that a young Queer person feels without having personally experienced the originating events. Epigenetic research lends intriguing support to the idea that trauma can become embodied across generations. Studies of survivors of extreme trauma have shown biological stress markers in their descendants. While the epigenetic transmission of Queer-specific trauma is not yet thoroughly studied, the principle from trauma science is clear: The body can carry echoes of historical oppression.[9] In Queer clients, those echoes might mingle with the physical stress imprints of racism, sexism, or other biases, weaving an embodied memory that is dense and complex.[10]

Attending to intersectionality in therapy means actively addressing the sociopolitical dimensions of a client's narrative. Therapists must educate themselves on how systems of oppression interact. For example, understanding the link between racism and body image is essential when working with Queer clients who struggle with their appearance. Clinical researchers have traced how contemporary beauty standards and fatphobia are rooted in racist ideologies that devalue Black bodies.[11] A Queer Black woman dealing with body shame may thus be fighting not only heteronormative expectations of femininity but also a legacy of racialized judgment in how she and her ancestors' bodies have been viewed. By bringing these connections into the open, therapy validates that her distress is not a personal failing but a reaction to oppressive narratives imposed on her. This validation is inherently healing; it moves the blame from the self to the social forces at play. It also expands the avenues for re-authoring the narrative: She can begin to script a story in which her body is reclaimed from those colonial and racial narratives. Similarly, Queer and trans people from conservative religious backgrounds may need to disentangle spiritual trauma from identity trauma. For example, a trans Latinx person raised in a strict faith community might carry internalized transphobia entwined with colonial-era religious dogmas about sin and purity. Effective narrative liberation will invite exploration of both aspects, perhaps incorporating culturally specific healing practices or community resources to address the unique blend of spiritual and gender-identity harm.

Intersectionality reminds us that healing itself must be contextualized. An intervention will likely fall flat if it ignores a client's cultural context. Consider somatic therapies: Shaking or trembling exercises (as in some trauma-release techniques) might be liberating for one client, but for another whose culture stigmatizes overt emotional expression, a different approach is needed. Being attuned to intersectional factors guides therapists in choosing and adapting techniques with cultural humility. Resmaa Menakem, in discussing racialized trauma, emphasizes that bodies of different backgrounds carry different pain and require different comforts; what soothes one nervous system might alarm another.[12] For instance, a Queer refugee who fled a country due to violently enforced homophobia may find safety in very gentle, private somatic practices at first (given their experience of surveillance and danger). In contrast, a more privileged Queer client might comfortably partake in loud, public expressions like a group dance. The intersection of migration trauma, cultural norms, and Queer identity demands an individualized approach to both somatic and narrative interventions.

An intersectional framework also challenges therapists to examine their positionality and biases continually. Working with Queer clients from diverse backgrounds entails being vigilant about not reenacting microaggressions or assumptions in the therapy space. Studies have documented that lesbian, gay, and bisexual clients often experience subtle microaggressions in counseling, even from well-intentioned therapists.[13] These might include assumptions about family composition, such as *Are you married? What does your wife do?* posed to a lesbian client, mispronouncing a cultural name, or minimizing experiences of racism under the guise of focusing only on sexuality. Such missteps can retraumatize clients by echoing the invalidation they face in society. Therefore, a harm reduction approach in an intersectional context means the therapist actively seeks to reduce harm from social oppression within therapy itself, using correct pronouns and names, inquiring about and respecting all facets of identity, acknowledging the realities of discrimination, and being open to feedback and education. Personal healing and social justice become intertwined. By helping clients name and navigate the converging forces in their lives, we empower them to rewrite their individual stories and situate those stories in a broader narrative of collective liberation.

The Power of Collective Storytelling in Queer Healing

While personal introspection is vital, many Queer individuals discover that certain wounds cannot fully mend in isolation. Healing is often a community process. Queer communities, forged in the shared fires of marginalization and resistance, have long been spaces where stories are exchanged, validated, and transformed. In narrative therapy, collective sharing can thicken preferred stories and dilute the power of problem-saturated ones. Telling one's story in a group of empathetic peers or hearing an elder recount how they survived and thrived offers a powerful antidote to the isolation and shame that trauma instills. Research has begun to confirm what Queer folks have intuitively known: Intergenerational storytelling can be an essential developmental resource, helping to build resilience and identity continuity in Queer communities.[14]

When younger Queer people hear the narratives of older generations about clandestine love in hostile times, the fight against AIDS, and the victories of past activism, they inherit not only trauma but also maps of hope. Community narratives offer templates for coping and for envisioning a future. When elders witness the openness and self-actualization of youth who grew up with slightly more acceptance, they also experience healing, seeing the fruits of their past struggles. This reciprocal exchange exemplifies how collective narrative work turns isolated personal tales into a shared legacy of perseverance and pride.

One format for community healing is expressive art group therapy specifically for Queer and trans individuals. Within a well-facilitated group, participants serve as both narrators and witnesses for each other. The simple act of speaking one's truth to attentive listeners can itself be liberating. As feminist philosopher Kelly Oliver asserts, being truly heard and "witnessed" is central to reclaiming one's subjectivity after trauma.[15]

In a Queer trauma group, when one person describes their experience of familial rejection or body dysphoria, others may nod in recognition, implicitly saying, *I see you, and I have been there too.* Such moments of recognition can undo the distorted belief that *I am alone in this suffering.* They also allow group members to externalize blame; rather than each individual seeing their pain as a private shame, the group can name the social injustices at fault, which converts personal pain into collective awareness and solidarity. This resembles what Paulo Freire described as "conscientization," the awakening of critical consciousness about oppression.[16] In practical terms, group members might engage in collective exercises: writing a communal letter to their younger Queer selves, or collaboratively re-writing a traditional fairy tale to have Queer protagonists, thereby re-authoring cultural narratives in real time. Shared creative acts reinforce that change is possible and that each person's narrative gains strength from the collective.

Beyond formal therapy groups, healing thrives in the organic collective practices of Queer communities, what we might call grassroots narrative work. Community art and performance have historically provided Queer people avenues to express and reshape their stories on their terms. For example, the ballroom culture pioneered by Black and Latinx Queer communities created spaces where chosen families vogue and dance, effectively co-authoring narratives of glamour, pride, and defiance that counteracted the racism, poverty, and homophobia outside the ballroom. Such spaces can be seen as what activists and therapists call temporary autonomous zones, pockets of liberation where mainstream rules are suspended and new identities can be enacted.[17] Similarly, community arts projects, such as a mural painted in a gay neighborhood commemorating victims of violence or a collaborative zine compiling coming-out stories, serve as collective narrative documents. They assert *We were here, we have suffered, and we have overcome.* Participating in these projects can be profoundly healing for contributors; the art-making process becomes a ritual of communal catharsis, and the final product stands as a public counter-narrative challenging stigma and erasure. Indeed, the art activism of groups like ACT UP during the AIDS crisis exemplifies how community narrative work not only heals but also demands societal change. Slogans like "Silence = Death" and the act of Queer folks taking to the streets with bold imagery (such as the pink triangle reclaimed from Holocaust-era persecution) transformed individual grief and rage into a loud collective story that altered public consciousness.

Another poignant grassroots example is the AIDS Memorial Quilt, which, during the height of the AIDS epidemic, stitched together thousands of fabric panels made by loved ones of those lost. Each panel told a personal story. They collectively covered entire city lawns, a patchwork narrative of love and grief that demanded the nation's attention and humanized stigmatized people. This massive communal art project not only helped survivors and community members mourn and heal, but it also shifted public perception by rendering the scale and individuality of the loss visible. Decades later, in the age of the internet, campaigns like the It Gets Better Project (where Queer adults share videos about overcoming their youthful struggles) continue this tradition of collective storytelling. By disseminating thousands of personal narratives of hope to Queer youth, such movements weave a safety net of communal wisdom: the message that no one is alone and that a brighter narrative is possible. Public narrative-sharing initiatives complement therapy by working at a cultural level. As more stories of Queer resilience and joy enter the mainstream, the more empowered individuals may feel to reimagine their own lives along those lines.

Community healing also intersects with social justice and advocacy. Liberating narratives at the personal level often galvanizes people to push for broader changes; conversely, activism can be therapeutic. Therapists practicing narrative liberation are increasingly mindful of engaging with the community context of their clients. This can mean helping clients connect with supportive networks as part of the treatment plan, recognizing that these communal experiences will reinforce the client's emerging liberatory narrative. Therapists can also step out of the office to partake in advocacy, joining Pride marches, volunteering at Queer centers, or educating policymakers, thereby working to dismantle the very systems that generated their clients' traumas. If a client sees their therapist actively standing up for Queer rights in the community, it can further validate their narrative of empowerment. For example, a non-binary client who struggles with healthcare discrimination might find it incredibly affirming if their therapist helps draft a respectful but firm complaint to a medical provider, or if the therapist can share knowledge of local clinicians known to be trans-friendly. Practical engagements show the client that their narrative of deserving care and dignity is echoed by real-world action.

There is also a place for structured collective narrative practices that bridge individual therapy and community life. Narrative therapy pioneers have developed methods like the "outsider witness" practice, where a client's story (with consent) is shared with a small audience of peers who then reflect on the strengths and values they heard in the story. This can be adapted in Queer support circles to significant effect, giving the storyteller the experience of multiple people actively reinforcing their preferred narrative. Another example is community storytelling events or healing circles, sometimes organized around specific identities. In these gatherings, storytelling is often paired with cultural rituals, perhaps a candlelight vigil to honor those lost to violence, followed by a round where each participant speaks from the heart. Such intentional blending of story and ritual in the community amplifies the therapeutic factors of solidarity and witness. Research in restorative justice and community dialogue indicates that when people speak and listen in a circle with agreed-upon guidelines of respect, power imbalances are addressed, and deeper understanding emerges.[18] In Queer narrative circles, this means that even differences within the group (for example, between older and younger members or between binary-identified and non-binary folks) can be navigated in a way that ensures everyone's story finds a place. The circle becomes a microcosm of the liberated world we are trying to build, where diversity is valued, power is shared, and each narrative is dignified.

Ultimately, community healing and collective narrative work remind us that the liberation of one story is tied to the liberation of all. When a Queer person transforms their narrative from one of victimhood to one of resilience, they shine a light that helps others do the same. Conversely, as communities challenge oppressive narratives publicly, individual members feel permission to rewrite their private stories. This synergy between the individual and the collective is the liberatory practice's heart. It is a revolution of small stories swelling into a chorus, a new social narrative in which Queer bodies are sites not of tragedy or shame but of strength, wisdom, and love.

Guiding Narrative Transformation in Queer Clients

A central tenet of narrative therapy is that how we story our lives strongly influences how we experience ourselves and what we believe is possible. Re-authoring is the therapeutic process of helping a client revise and expand their narrative, especially in ways that challenge limiting or oppressive plots. For Queer clients, narrative re-authoring can be a radical act of liberation. They often come into therapy with stories that have been heavily influenced by dominant heteronormative discourses, stories of being "wrong," "sinful," "broken," or "undeserving" because of who they are. These narratives might not be explicitly stated, but they manifest in feelings of shame, internalized homophobia/transphobia, or a sense of disconnect from one's own body. The task of re-authoring is to externalize one's negative narratives, such as seeing "shame" as a product of societal prejudice rather than a truth about oneself, and to co-create new narratives that foreground one's strengths, values, and authentic identity. In practice, this could involve a client identifying "unique outcomes," moments in their life when the oppressive story did not hold, and building on them. For example, a transgender man might recall a childhood memory of feeling pure joy when he secretly wore his brother's clothes, a moment that contradicts the dominant narrative that "something is wrong with me." The therapist can help him richly describe that memory and explore its meaning (perhaps it shows his resourcefulness and inner knowledge of self), then begin to thicken this alternative storyline of self-knowledge and resilience. Over time, these once-sparse alternative narratives gain detail and emotional weight, becoming viable new foundations for identity.

Narrative re-authoring is inherently a social justice intervention because it challenges the internalized voice of oppression. In the Queer context, re-authoring often means explicitly naming and critiquing the social narratives that have harmed the client. A client might externalize depression as "the weight of heteronormativity" or envision their anxiety as a "protective guard" that appeared because the world has been unsafe for them. This de-personalization of problems, a hallmark of narrative therapy, creates breathing room for self-compassion and critical awareness. It echoes Freire's idea of developing a critical consciousness: The client comes to see, for instance, that their sense of worthlessness is not an innate truth but the outcome of years of societal rejection. From this new vantage point, the client can author a counter-narrative. Perhaps instead of *I am unlovable,* the emerging narrative becomes *I have survived in a world that did not always love me, and that survival is proof of my worth and strength.* This shift from an oppressed narrative to a liberation narrative is the psychological equivalent of coming out of a narrow closet into a vast open field. The client's story now accommodates pride, resistance, and community connection where there was isolation and stigma before.

Effective re-authoring with Queer clients pays attention to the language of the story. Language is political; the words used to describe identity or experience carry societal connotations. Part of liberating one's narrative may involve reclaiming language, as in the proud use of the once-derogatory term "Queer" or inventing new terms for novel experiences. It can also include rejecting labels that do not fit. For example, an asexual non-binary client might re-author their story to assert that their lack of sexual attraction is not a defect (as a society might insinuate) but a valid identity; they may choose metaphors of fullness and self-containment rather than the standard narrative of "lacking" something. Metaphors and creative writing can play a decisive role here. Therapists often encourage clients to write letters, perhaps a "letter from your future self" or a letter to the people who have hurt you, to articulate the re-authored narrative in a concrete form. Using metaphor and imagery in art helps bypass internal censors and tap into more profound truths.[19] Individuals who have long felt alien in their skin might describe their journey as a phoenix rising from the ashes or a butterfly emerging from a cocoon, metaphors that reframe transformation as natural and beautiful. Such images stick in the mind and can be drawn on in moments of doubt, reinforcing the new narrative.

Crucially, narrative re-authoring for Queer clients must be paced and guided by the client's readiness, a principle in line with harm reduction. A therapist steeped in allyship might be eager for their client to embrace an empowering narrative. However, pushing that story can feel disingenuous or even invalidating if the client is not there yet. It is essential to first witness the old narrative with empathy and acknowledge how it formed and may have served the client in some way. For instance, *I will never find love* might have been a protective response to repeated rejections; simply telling the client to believe *I am lovable* without addressing the pain underneath may ring hollow. Harm reduction in narrative work means nurturing change without forcing it. As Kuhfuß highlights, therapy should honor clients' multiple truths and support them in moving toward a more empowering story at their own pace. Re-authoring often begins with minor edits, not a total rewrite overnight.[20] The client might start by acknowledging one aspect of themself in a kinder light, gradually building up to broader self-acceptance. These subtle narrative shifts accumulate, reducing the harm of self-stigma and replacing it with self-compassion and pride.

In re-authoring, witnesses and audiences to the new story are essential. Sharing a re-authored narrative with trusted others, be it a partner, a friend, or a Queer support group, and getting affirmative feedback can reinforce it. This is where our previous discussion of community healing dovetails with individual narrative work. A story finds its full power when it is told and received. Queer communities often celebrate re-authored narratives in rituals like name-change ceremonies for trans individuals or "second birthdays," marking the anniversary of coming out. These communal acknowledgments serve as milestones that say the new story is real and honored by others. Each time someone reflects on a client's liberated narrative, *I see how far you have come,* it gains solidity.

Narrative re-authoring also opens up future horizons. It is not just about reinterpreting the past but about altering the trajectory of one's story into the future. Queer theorist José Esteban Muñoz speaks of Queer futurity, the notion that true freedom for Queer people is always something being imagined and strived for, a "not-yet-here" potential.[21] In therapy, when a Queer person re-authors their narrative, they are actively engaging in Queer futurity on a personal level. They are projecting a self that can exist and flourish in the world, often in ways with no past precedent in their family or community. A young non-binary person may craft a narrative of their future where they create the family of choice they never had, or a middle-aged gay man might reimagine his later life not as lonely aging but as full of creative community endeavors. The new narrative acts as a beacon, guiding present decisions. Visioning a livable, fulfilling future is a profound protective factor against despair. It is one reason narrative work is so tied to hope. We instill a forward-looking momentum by helping clients articulate who they are now and who they are becoming. Each step they take, whether applying for a job they once thought impossible as an out Queer person, pursuing a healthy relationship, or simply dressing in clothes that align with their gender, becomes part of their story of growth rather than a "risky" anomaly.

Narrative re-authoring empowers Queer individuals to step out of the scripts written for them by others and to write their own. It transforms phrases like *I cannot* into *I choose* and *I am broken* into *I am whole.* This is not to suggest that the end product is a saccharine or unrealistically optimistic story. On the contrary, liberatory narratives are richly complex and realistic. They acknowledge hardship and injustice, but these elements are framed within a larger story of survival, meaning-making, and pride. The client emerges not as a passive character to whom life "happened" but as an active protagonist, even an author, of their life. Reclaiming authorship is deeply political for Queer people, who have historically been denied the right to tell their own stories. As one narrative therapy proverb goes: *The person is not the problem; the problem is the problem, and the person is the author of their story.* In liberating their narrative, Queer individuals redefine themselves from the inside out, a necessary step toward the kind of embodied freedom and authenticity that we have been exploring throughout this work.

Expressive Therapies in Queer Narrative Transformation

Expressive therapies operate on the principle that creative expression can bypass the limitations of ordinary talk, accessing deeper layers of emotion and bodily knowledge.[22] One key benefit of expressive art therapy is its ability to facilitate embodiment gently and indirectly. Instead of being asked to verbally describe their feelings about their body, a client might be invited to sculpt an abstract form that represents how they experience themself or to draw their body as a landscape. For instance, a non-binary client sketches themself as a tree with tangled roots and a sky-reaching crown, externalizing their feelings of being grounded yet aspiring for freedom. The therapist and client can then explore the image: *What do the tangled roots need, perhaps untangling or water (nurturance)? What does the open sky symbolize to you?* Through metaphor, the client often finds it easier to discuss vulnerable aspects of their relationship with their body. The process creates a slight distance from pain (since it is happening "in the artwork"), paradoxically making it safer to approach that pain. Moreover, translating bodily experiences into art engages sensorimotor processes that aid integration: As the client uses their hands, sees colors and shapes, hears sounds, or feels their body moving, multiple brain regions activate in concert. Neuropsychological research suggests that such multisensory engagement can help trauma survivors integrate memories and emotions that were previously fragmented or wordless.[23] In this way, expressive art acts as a bridge between the nonverbal memory of the body and the conscious re-authoring of narrative.

Different art modalities offer distinct pathways to liberation. Visual art therapy, such as painting, drawing, or collage, yields tangible representations of the client's internal world. These artifacts can be revisited over time, allowing clients to "see" their progress or recurring themes. A series of self-portraits made throughout therapy, for example, might evolve from dark, chaotic scribbles to more coherent and vibrant images as the client's narrative shifts toward self-acceptance. Such progress need not be linear or directly representational; even color choice or line quality changes can signify narrative change.[24] Visual art can also challenge internalized images of the body. In a supportive exercise, a therapist might ask a client to draw their body outline on a large piece of paper (a form of body mapping) and then fill it with symbols of both pain and strength: maybe jagged lines where there are scars, but also bright patches where the client feels pride or pleasure. This external map of the body becomes a site of exploration and dialogue. Clients often discover that how they depict their body on paper is more compassionate and nuanced than the harsh mental image they carry, an essential step toward liberating the real body from false narratives of "ugliness" or "wrongness."

Dance and movement are also avenues toward liberation. Traumatic experiences and social oppression can leave Queer individuals disconnected from their physical selves, moving gingerly, hunching to avoid attention, or even feeling estranged from the body's sensations. In dance/movement therapy, clients are encouraged to let their body speak through motion. This might start with subtle gestures: Perhaps the client sways while seated or experiments with the feeling of pressing their feet firmly into the ground. Over time, as safety grows, movement can become more expansive. The act of dancing freely can be radically liberating for someone whose movements have been policed or shamed (imagine a gender-nonconforming child who was told not to "sway his hips" now finding joy in swaying unapologetically in a therapy studio). The movement also directly engages the nervous system's capacity for regulation. Rhythmic motion and synchronized actions (even something as simple as the client and therapist snapping their fingers or clapping in time together) can bring the client's arousal down from hypervigilance or up from dissociation, steering them toward a window of functionality where healing happens.[25] In group settings, collective movement, like a circle of Queer adults moving in unison to a drumbeat, reinforces community and the feeling of "moving together" through shared struggles. This physical synchrony can foster profound belonging, embodying the idea that we are all together. In a Queer context, that sense of solidarity in motion directly counters the isolating bodily shame many have felt.

Music taps into the deep emotional resonance of sound. Many Queer people have personal anthems or songs that have buoyed them during difficult times; tapping into this, a therapist might explore which songs or sounds empower the client and why. Songwriting can be a potent technique; for instance, a bisexual client might write lyrics about claiming their *whole* identity ("not half of anything") and set it to the melody of a favorite song, effectively re-authoring their narrative in musical form.[26] When sung communally, those personalized verses turn into a celebration of each member's journey. Rhythmic drumming or heartbeat imitations in music can also help clients release anger or grief that words cannot reach, offering a cathartic reclamation of voice and pulse. For clients who find silence comforting, instrumental music or ambient soundscapes can create a safe auditory atmosphere in which they can relax and feel held. The beauty of music is that it connects directly to emotions and physiology, slowing the breath, relaxing muscle tension, or energizing the spirit, thus aligning the body with the emerging positive narrative.

Similarly, drama and role-play can enable Queer clients to experiment with stories. Many have had to perform restrictive roles in real life (hiding their true gender, playing the "perfect child" to avoid rejection, etc.). In therapy, they can play new roles: the hero, the nurturer, the rebel, the beloved. A drama technique might guide a client through an empty-chair exercise where the client speaks as their Proud Self, addressing their Ashamed Self, effectively acting out an internal dialogue and allowing the Proud Self to take the stage. This kind of externalization through performance can unstick aspects of the narrative that feel intractable. It also harnesses the inherently performative nature of identity highlighted by Judith Butler; since gender and social roles involve performance, consciously performing one's liberatory narrative in the therapy space (even symbolically) can help solidify it.[27] Some clients literally script and act out pivotal scenes of their lives but with new endings, a form of therapeutic role-play that lets them experience mastery or closure. They might reenact confronting a bully but practice responding with confidence and boundary-setting this time. Witnessing and validating these enactments, the therapist (and possibly group members) provides audience feedback reinforcing the new narrative: *We see you as strong and worthy.* The embodied experience of such role-play lingers in the body's memory, providing a rehearsal for real-life situations.

Because expressive art therapy supports an affirmative and client-centered approach, the client is inherently positioned as the creator and as the expert in their experience. Peuser emphasizes that creative arts therapists working with Queer populations should remain flexible and attuned to clients' unique cultural expressions, whether that is drawing on drag performance aesthetics or integrating Queer icons and media into therapeutic art projects.[28] The goal is to make the therapeutic canvas or stage a mirror of the client's multifaceted identity, where all parts of them have permission to exist and create.

Expressive therapies are not only about expressing pain; they are equally about expressing joy, desire, and hope. Liberating Queer body narratives means reducing trauma symptoms and also expanding capacity for pleasure and creativity in the body. Through dance, a Queer person may rediscover the sensual joy in their movements; through art, they may celebrate their body with colors and shapes that feel like a homecoming. Positive embodied experiences are crucial for counteracting trauma. They give the body new memories to hold, memories of Pride marches danced, of communal songs sung, of the quiet focus of painting something that matters. Such experiences get woven into the narrative as well, ensuring that the Queer story is not defined solely by struggle but also by resilience, artfulness, and the defiant happiness of self-expression. In effect, expressive art therapy helps write the body's poetry into the personal narrative, those metaphorical lines and verses that capture the beauty of Queer existence. When the body can be a source of creativity and pleasure again, it is a strong sign that the narrative of liberation has taken root.

By practicing embodied rituals, Queer individuals reclaim their body moment by moment. By centering intersectionality, they contextualize their pain and resistance within broader histories, turning shame into insight and isolation into solidarity. Through community and collective storytelling, their voice gains strength in chorus, echoing through intergenerational trauma to break long-held silences. Through narrative re-authoring, they wield the pen of identity, revising harmful scripts and writing new chapters filled with agency and pride. Expressive art therapies tap into the body's wisdom and creativity, accessing forms of knowing and release beyond words. In a world that still imposes myriad harms on Queer and trans bodies, the work of liberating narratives remains urgent. It is a form of resistance and self-preservation as much as a path to individual fulfillment. The sociopolitical dimensions of Queer healing mean that every personal breakthrough has ripples: A Queer person who finds self-love may become an advocate who helps change their community, and a community that embraces liberatory practices nurtures the next generation's ability to thrive. Narrative liberation is, ultimately, a continuous and collective journey. It asks us, as Audre Lorde urged, that we transform silence into language and action, and that we do so grounded in the wisdom of our bodies and the richness of our communities.[29] As therapists our role is to support this unfolding, to listen deeply, to witness without judgment, to offer tools of expression, and to stand beside Queer individuals as they author narratives that honor their truth. In liberating the narrative, we move closer to a world where every body, in all its Queerness and complexity, can tell their story without fear.

Case Example: The Liberated Narrative Through Art

The interplay of trauma, disordered eating, and gender dysphoria can leave people with complex narratives of pain, loss, and resilience. This case study examines the therapeutic journey of an AFAB (assigned female at birth) non-binary individual (they/them) in their fifties who is married to a cisgender man, with both partners identifying as bisexual. Their story is one of recovery from atypical anorexia, exercise abuse, and diet pill abuse; it is also a story marked by a long history of complex post-traumatic stress disorder stemming from early childhood abuse, painful estrangement from extended family due to unresolved familial trauma, and a life that included the responsibility of caretaking for ill grandparents. Despite these challenges, the client's resilience shines through, as they have forged a successful career as a nurse and academic, holding a PhD in nursing and working in a community mental and medical health agency.

Expressive art therapy has been a powerful tool for the client in their journey. They used it to confront and transform the challenges they faced, particularly in navigating gender dysphoria related to their fat body (per the client's description of themself). This dysphoria is deeply intertwined with societal narratives that dictate narrow definitions of beauty, body size, and gender. The client's transformation of old department store mannequins into powerful artistic expressions is a testament to their proactive approach to healing. These art pieces have evolved into potent messages of political resistance against cis-heteronormative patriarchy while also serving as vibrant celebrations of body euphoria and affirmations of the intricate complexities found in the Queer body narrative.

In their early years, they internalized societal expectations about gender and body image while grappling with their emerging sense of identity. Over time, these early experiences contributed to feelings of isolation and dysphoria, particularly as they navigated a world that often-imposed strict boundaries for femininity and beauty. Now in their fifties, the client has embraced their non-binary identity and rejected the limited narratives about what a body should look like. The client is married to a cisgender man; their relationship is characterized by a strong mutual commitment to personal growth and social justice, with their shared bisexuality providing a framework for exploring the fluidity of desire and identity. This dynamic has profoundly influenced the client's creative and political work, even as the couple has faced external pressures from a society that frequently imposes binary norms on relationships, sexuality, and gender expression.

Academically, the client is a beacon of achievement. Their work in community mental and medical health agencies has been instrumental in advocating for marginalized populations and addressing systemic inequities in healthcare. Their professional identity is a source of immense pride and resilience, representing personal achievement and a commitment to healing underserved communities. Balancing a demanding career with ongoing personal healing, the client has learned to integrate their lived experiences with their professional role. Their academic and clinical work often intersects with their journey, enriching their understanding of the interplay between trauma, identity, and health. This dual role has allowed them to become a role model within their community, demonstrating that personal transformation is possible and can catalyze broader societal change.

The client's history is marred by early childhood abuse, which left deep emotional scars. Both physical and psychological abuse contributed to the development of complex PTSD, embedding a pervasive sense of mistrust, fear, and difficulty with self-regulation and boundary-setting. Over the years, the client has diligently worked through many layers of this trauma in therapy, though remnants of those early wounds continue to influence their self-perception and relationships. Family dynamics further complicated the client's struggles with identity and trust. Their extended family's persistent denial of the childhood abuse, along with an inability to acknowledge or validate those traumatic events, led to a painful estrangement. This rejection compounded the client's trauma and instilled a long-term sense of isolation and abandonment, leading them to seek solace and validation from other sources, such as their professional community and, eventually, Queer social networks.

During a particularly challenging stage in adulthood, the client assumed the caretaker role for their ailing grandparents. Although this role was deeply rooted in love and a sense of duty, it added another complexity to their identity. The responsibility of caregiving often necessitated sacrificing personal needs, and the emotional burden of witnessing the decline of loved ones further complicated the client's recovery journey. Nonetheless, this experience also instilled a profound sense of empathy and resilience that later informed their clinical work and personal healing.

The client's recovery journey has been particularly challenging due to a long history of disordered eating behaviors. Unlike classical anorexia nervosa, the client's experience is best characterized as atypical anorexia, marked by restrictive eating patterns that did not necessarily conform to the typical body mass index criteria. A pattern of exercise abuse and a dangerous reliance on diet pills compounded their struggles. These self-destructive behaviors were an attempt to exert control over their body in response to feelings of dysphoria and internalized shame. Recovery was far from linear; the client underwent multiple cycles of dieting, over-exercising, and the hazardous use of weight-control pills. This pattern, closely intertwined with their gender dysphoria, reflected a constant tension between the desire to conform to societal expectations and a simultaneous rejection of those very standards. The recovery process involved dismantling these harmful behaviors and learning to appreciate the body in all its complexity, recognizing its inherent beauty and worth.

The lasting impact of childhood abuse manifests as complex PTSD, characterized by emotional dysregulation, intrusive memories, and difficulties in forming secure attachments. These symptoms became a constant undercurrent in the client's life, influencing their relationships and how they navigated social situations. Episodes of hypervigilance, dissociation, and chronic feelings of shame and guilt would often surface during periods of stress, impeding the client's ability to engage with life fully. Therapeutic interventions targeting C-PTSD required a multifaceted approach that integrated trauma-informed care with strategies for emotional regulation and self-compassion. Over time, the client's work in therapy allowed them to acknowledge the roots of their trauma and begin the arduous process of healing, despite setbacks and the need for ongoing support.

Their gender dysphoria was a significant source of distress, mainly as it related to their curvy, fat body. Societal messages that devalue larger bodies and prescribe narrow definitions of gender expression contributed to deep-seated insecurities. The client's internal conflict was not solely about physical appearance; it was also about how their body was perceived and validated within both cis-normative and Queer spaces. For many years, the client felt trapped between two conflicting narratives: on one side, the dominant cultural expectation that equates thinness with beauty, and on the other, a Queer subversion of these norms through body positivity and liberation. Their journey involved a rigorous process of challenging both internalized fatphobia and the rigid gender binaries that dictated how they should look and feel. Ultimately, the acceptance and celebration of their body became a pivotal aspect of their healing process, leading to a transformative experience of body euphoria.

An intersectional framework was essential in addressing the many layers of the client's identity, which encompassed their non-binary gender identity, traumatic past, disordered eating behaviors, and professional roles. This approach provided a comprehensive understanding of how overlapping systems of oppression and privilege shaped their experiences. The integration of Queer liberation as a political and cultural stance offered the client a robust conceptual foundation for their therapeutic journey. Rejecting cis-heteronormative norms and embracing diverse expressions of identity became central themes in their path toward self-acceptance. By combining Queer theory with trauma-informed care and expressive arts therapy, the intervention was designed not only to alleviate symptoms but also to empower the client both politically and personally.

Expressive art therapy was a transformative tool for the client. Creative expression provided a means to externalize their deeply held emotions, transform trauma, and reclaim the body as a source of strength and resistance. The process of working with art became a language, a nonverbal dialogue that allowed them to communicate experiences that were otherwise too difficult to articulate. Central to this client's creative process was their innovative use of old department store mannequins. Once emblematic of rigid, idealized beauty and consumerist conformity, the mannequins were repurposed as blank canvases ripe for transformation. In reclaiming these objects, the client challenged the foundations upon which traditional beauty standards were built, subverting the symbolism embedded in their original form.

To deepen the client's engagement with expressive arts, I deliberately cultivated a brave space and established Queer sanctuary. In practice, a brave space invited the client to take interpersonal and intrapsychic risks, experimenting with unfamiliar materials, confronting internalized norms, and voicing emergent stories, while trusting that their disclosures would be met with respect and confidentiality. Simultaneously, framing the studio as a Queer sanctuary signaled an explicit rejection of cis-heteronormativity and affirmed the validity of all non-binary and Queer expressions. Within this dual container, the client felt empowered to dwell in tension, tolerate ambiguity, and witness their own unfolding without self-criticism. This environment not only fostered the emotional safety necessary for vulnerability in art-making but also reinforced a collective ethos of resilience and solidarity, thereby amplifying the transformative potential of the mannequin interventions and other creative modalities.

The mannequin project was multilayered and evolved over months of creative exploration. Initially, the client encountered the mannequins as relics of a commercial past, objects crafted to embody the ideals of a beauty industry obsessed with perfection and uniformity. With their unyielding, faceless forms, the mannequins served as stark reminders of the pressure to conform, their cold surfaces reflecting the harsh judgment of a society that prized an unattainable standard. But as the client began to interact with these objects in the controlled, nurturing space of expressive art therapy, they discovered the potential to transform these symbols of oppression into vessels of liberation.

Through a series of intimate, emotionally charged sessions, the client started by dismantling the traditional image of the mannequin. With gentle, deliberate strokes, they removed layers of synthetic material, each fragment representing an internalized belief or a painful memory tied to the ideals of beauty that had once caused immense suffering. This deconstruction was not a destructive act but rather a process of peeling away layers of cultural conditioning to reveal a raw, unfiltered core. In this space, authentic self-expression could emerge. Deconstructing the mannequin became a ritual of liberation, a symbolic shedding of the old self and the external expectations that had long dictated the client's sense of worth.

As the client progressed in their work, the process evolved into reconstruction. With each new session, fragments of the old mannequin were reassembled in unexpected, creative ways. The client began introducing new materials, vivid fabrics, reflective surfaces, and elements drawn from nature, symbolizing the reclaiming of their narrative. These additions were not random; they were imbued with personal significance, each piece carefully chosen to represent an aspect of the client's journey toward self-acceptance. The interplay of colors, textures, and shapes on the reimagined mannequin reflected the complexity of the client's identity, a tapestry woven from threads of resilience, pain, and ultimate triumph.

Through this process, the mannequin transformed from a cold, impersonal object into a dynamic, living work of art that embodied the client's internal metamorphosis (see Figures 13, 14, and 15).

An intense, ongoing internal dialogue accompanied the transformation. As the client manipulated and reworked the mannequins, they engaged in meditative self-reflection. Long periods of silence during the creative sessions allowed the client to listen deeply to their inner voice, a voice that societal norms and traumatic experiences had long suppressed. In these moments of stillness, the client began to experience their body as a site of memory and possibility, where each brushstroke and each cut of fabric carried the weight of both past wounds and emerging hope. The creative act became an

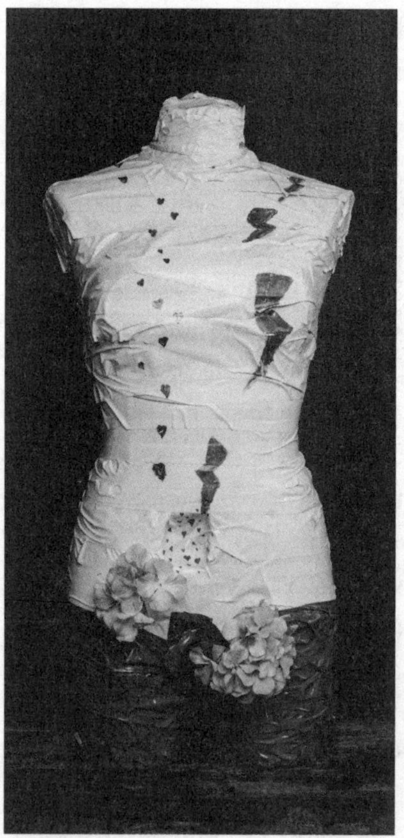

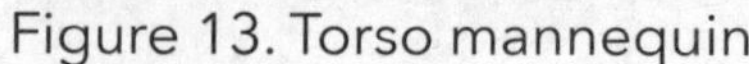

Figure 13. Torso mannequin

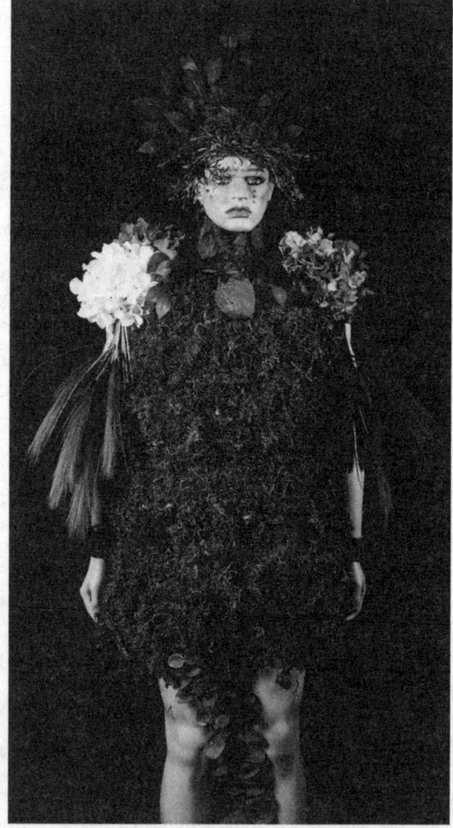

Figure 14. Full body mannequin

embodied experience in which the client could physically feel the tension and the eventual release as the old layers gave way to new expressions of self. This was not merely art-making but a profound self-rediscovery, reclaiming the body and mind as integral parts of a holistic identity.

Over time, the client's work began to garner attention beyond the therapy room: The reimagined mannequins were displayed in community gatherings and local exhibitions. The public presentations of these artworks sparked conversations about the very nature of beauty, the politics of representation, and the possibility of healing through art. For many viewers, the pieces served as a mirror reflecting their struggles and aspirations, a call to re-examine internalized beliefs about gender and body image. The

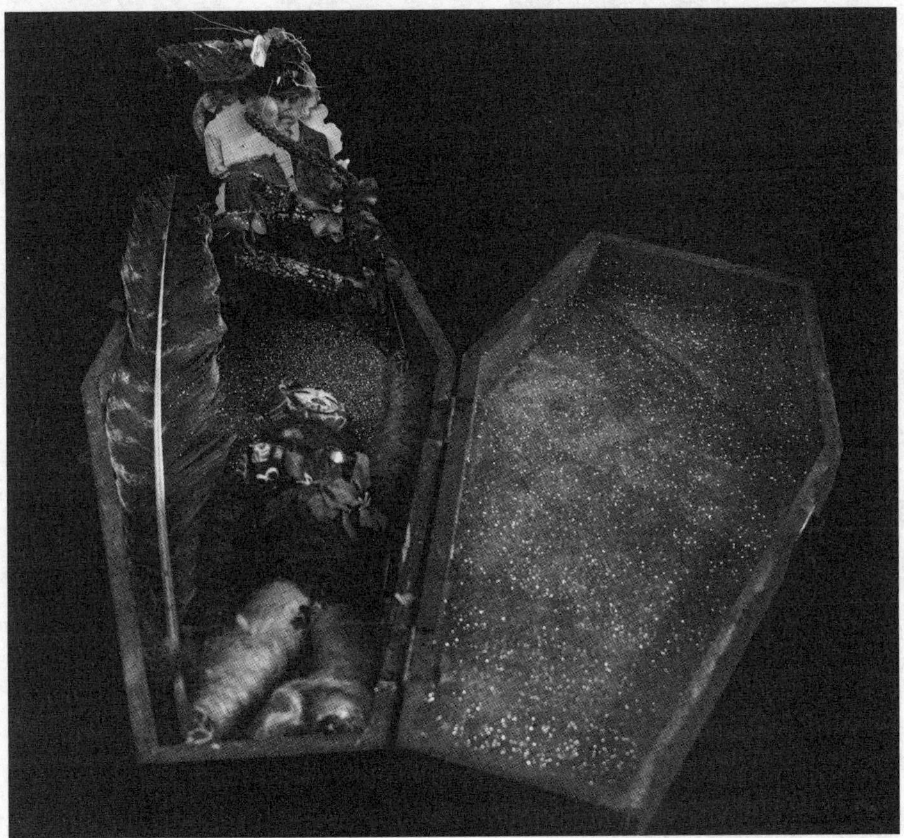

Figure 15. Coffin sculpture

client's art resonated deeply with those who had long felt marginalized by rigid societal standards, and the exhibitions became spaces where conversations about Queer liberation and body positivity could flourish openly and vulnerably.

In sharing their work with a broader audience, the client discovered that the creative process had far-reaching implications. Once transformed into vivid, multidimensional sculptures, the mannequins had transcended their original role as personal artifacts; they had become symbols of collective resistance. The art served as an invitation for other people to explore their narratives of pain and hope, to question the norms that had once confined them, and to imagine new ways of being that celebrated diversity and authenticity. This communal aspect of expressive art therapy deeply validated the client. It reinforced the notion that healing is not a solitary endeavor but a shared journey that thrives on connection, empathy, and the collective reimagining of cultural narratives.

The process of creating and sharing these artworks also had a profound impact on the client's internal landscape. Interacting with the transformed mannequins reinforced a growing sense of agency and self-worth. The client began to see their body as a repository of strength, memory, and beauty. The once-dreaded image of the curvy, fat body gradually transformed into a powerful symbol of resistance against a culture that had long attempted to dictate its value. The artistic process allowed the client to celebrate every curve and contour as an essential part of their identity, which was complex, multifaceted, and inherently valuable.

To deepen the client's internalization of both brave space and Queer sanctuary, the therapeutic setting was carefully structured along several interwoven dimensions. At the outset, therapist and client collaboratively generated a set of relational agreements, ground rules that acknowledged power imbalances, honored confidentiality, and named potential triggers. By co-authoring these guidelines, the client claimed agency over the parameters of their vulnerability. In turn, violating these agreements (whether by therapist, client, or even the materials themselves, such as a sharp tool in a sculpture activity) became an invitation to pause, reflect, and repair, rather than a source of shame or retreat.

Entering the art studio each session was framed as a ritual movement from the hyper-regulated "outside world" into a purposefully deregulated, Queer-affirming zone. A simple ritual, ringing a small bell or laying down a sprig of lavender at the studio door, served as a collective signal that normative constraints were being left behind. This transition ceremony not only demarcated the physical space but also primed the client's nervous system for creative risk-taking and embodied exploration. The studio became the embodiment of Queer sanctuary, spaces that hold deep meaning, preservation of culture, and rest.

Beyond mannequins, a curated palette of textures, colors, and forms was made available that explicitly broke from gender-binary conventions: iridescent fabrics, neon pigments, modular foam shapes, and found-object assemblage materials. Each of these "queer tools" carried an invitation to experiment with embodied identities, stretching, layering, and adorning the mannequin bodies in ways that resisted categorization. I encouraged journaling or spoken reflection on how each material felt "in" their body, creating a somatic feedback loop that reinforced bodily autonomy.

When the client felt ready, elements of their creative process were shared in small, carefully screened peer-support gatherings composed of other Queer and non-binary artists in therapy. These witnessing circles modeled collective care: Each participant offered "radical affirmation" feedback, naming strengths, curiosities, and transformative moments they observed in each other's work. This communal witnessing further solidified the container, expanding it into a wider Queer sanctuary network that amplified the client's sense of belonging to a living lineage of creative resistance. Maintaining a brave space requires continual reflection on relational dynamics. I committed to regular debriefs, checking in not only on the client's experience of the space (e.g., "What felt possible, and what felt too unsafe?") but also on their own positioning and potential enactment of norms. This reflexive posture ensured that the Queer sanctuary remained dynamic and responsive, rather than ossifying into a new set of prescriptive expectations.

By layering these strategies, co-created norms, transitional rituals, radical materials, communal witnessing, and ongoing reflexivity, the therapeutic milieu became both a brave space for risk-taking and a Queer sanctuary for belonging. In this richly held container, the client could reclaim creative agency, re-author their relationship with their body, and discover new modes of resilience that carried far beyond the walls of the studio.

As their creative journey continued, the expressive art therapy sessions expanded in scope. The client began experimenting with collaborative projects, inviting peers and members of the community to participate in the creative process. In these sessions, collective creativity served as a healing tool and a platform for activism. The group dynamics fostered an environment in which ideas flowed freely, and the energy of communal expression amplified the impact of each contribution. The act of reimagining the mannequins evolved into a shared celebration of diversity, showing the power of art to bridge personal and political divides. The integration of expressive art therapy into the client's broader therapeutic regimen catalyzed a holistic transformation in all facets of their life. The client's newfound confidence and clarity professionally enriched their work as a nurse and academic. The insights gained through creative expression deepened their understanding of trauma, gender, and the healing potential of art, knowledge that they enthusiastically shared with colleagues and students. This integration of personal and professional growth bolstered the client's sense of empowerment and inspired others facing similar struggles. Their academic contributions began to reflect a nuanced understanding of the intersections between creative expression and mental health, influencing policy discussions and educational programs in their field.

The personal ripple effects of the art therapy work extended into every corner of the client's life. The client discovered that as they became more comfortable with their own body and identity, they were able to connect with others on a deeper level. Relationships once strained by internalized shame and societal judgment began flourishing in an environment of mutual understanding and acceptance. The act of sharing their journey, through both conversation and art, became a liberating experience that opened doors to new relationships and communities. The creative process had mended internal fractures and served as a bridge to a more compassionate, interconnected world.

The client's ongoing engagement with expressive art therapy yielded new insights and breakthroughs in the following years. They maintained a rigorous practice of documenting their creative process through detailed journals, photography, and reflective writing, ensuring that each stage of transformation was captured as part of a living archive of their journey. This continuous documentation provided a rich resource for personal reflection and broader advocacy efforts, reinforcing that healing is an ongoing, dynamic process. The records of their artistic evolution became a testament to the transformative potential of creative expression, a source of inspiration for others, and a blueprint for those seeking to reclaim their narratives. The client's work with the mannequins ultimately transcended the realm of therapy and entered the sphere of cultural activism. Their art was featured in public installations, community art shows, and even local media segments highlighting innovative healing and self-expression approaches. In public forums, the transformed mannequins served as rallying points for discussions about body positivity, Queer liberation, and the urgent need to dismantle oppressive cultural norms. The client became an active voice in these dialogues, using their personal narrative and creative work as a platform to advocate for broader societal change. Their transformation journey resonated with many people, sparking a movement that celebrated diversity and challenged the status quo in tangible, visible ways.

Throughout every stage of this journey, the client deepened their awareness of the interconnectedness between personal healing and collective empowerment. The process of transforming the mannequins, which began as a personal act of rebellion, evolved into a broader cultural statement. It underscored the belief that art, in its most honest form, has the power to heal, question, and transform. The vibrant sculptures that emerged from the once-sterile forms of department store mannequins bore witness to this truth. They stood as bold declarations that external standards do not dictate beauty, and that beauty is an inherent quality that radiates from the courage to be oneself in all the messy, magnificent complexity that life entails.

The evolution of the client's creative practice was marked by moments of profound revelation. In the quiet intensity of the studio, as the client carefully reassembled fragments of the past into something new and meaningful, an overwhelming sense of liberation washed over them. The act of creation became a ritual of renewal, where each piece of reclaimed material and every new artistic addition symbolized a reclaiming of self. This journey was not without its moments of struggle; there were times when the weight of past trauma threatened to overwhelm the creative spirit. With each setback, however, came a deeper commitment to the transformative power of art.

In reflecting on this expansive journey, it is clear that the expressive art therapy process, embodied so vividly in reimagining department store mannequins, was not merely a method of artistic expression but a revolutionary act of self-determination. The client's ability to take an object once steeped in consumer culture and transform it into an emblem of resistance, beauty, and hope demonstrates the transformative power of creativity. This process allowed them to challenge the confines of societal norms and to assert a narrative in which their body, identity, and experiences were valid and worthy of celebration. The legacy of this creative journey is one of enduring empowerment. As the client continues to share their work with diverse audiences, the impact of their transformation ripples outward, offering others the courage to challenge their own limiting beliefs. The mannequins, now replete with the colors, textures, and symbols of a hard-won victory over internalized oppression, serve as permanent reminders that healing is possible even in the face of overwhelming adversity. In every meticulously reconstructed detail and expressive brushstroke, a story of resilience unfolds, one that speaks to the indomitable spirit of those who dare to reclaim their narratives and redefine beauty on their own terms.

Ultimately, the legacy of this work is measured not only by the striking visual impact of the transformed mannequins but also by the profound, lasting changes they have catalyzed within the client's life and those touched by their story. Through art, the client has discovered that healing is not a destination but a continuous journey of creation, exploration, and renewal. This journey transforms pain into power, isolation into connection, and doubt into a profound celebration of the self.

Continuous Liberation and Healing

Queer liberation is not a one-time event but an ongoing process, a continuous journey that evolves with each generation and each personal narrative. In the context of healing from body-based trauma, continuous liberation means that Queer individuals repeatedly engage in practices that reclaim their bodies and identities, reaffirming their freedom in the face of ongoing societal pressures. Liberation unfolds in moments big and small: private therapeutic breakthroughs, collective celebrations, and daily acts of resistance. Crucially, this journey is both personal and collective. Each individual's growth can ripple outward to the community and culture, and your role as an academic, therapist, or practitioner is integral to this process. Grounded in our bodies' wisdom and communities' richness, continuous liberation acknowledges that healing and freedom require persistent effort, courage, and creativity. In liberation Queer and trans people can safely explore identity, embodiment, and creative expression without the usual constraints, thereby generating new possibilities for living. Liberation, in this sense, is not a fixed endpoint but an ongoing praxis: a cycle of action and reflection where theory, creativity, and lived experience inform each other continuously.

Healing from trauma, especially for Queer and trans individuals, demands a holistic theoretical framework. Somatic theory, expressive arts, Queer theory, and harm reduction each offer crucial insights, and together they form a comprehensive foundation for continuous liberation. Somatic theory posits that the body is central to processing trauma:

Experiences of oppression and violence are not just stored in memory but are also held in muscle tension, posture, breath, and the nervous system. The saying "the body keeps the score" captures how unhealed trauma can manifest physically. Indeed, research on the autonomic nervous system shows that our bodies retain responses to past threats. Somatic approaches like somatic experiencing and sensorimotor psychotherapy aim to release these embodied stress responses, facilitating trauma integration and nervous system regulation.[30] Within Queer trauma healing, a somatic lens validates that the body itself narrates part of the story. Bodily sensations, a racing heart, a choked throat, or a collapsed posture can signal internalized shame or fear, while shifts in those sensations (a deep breath, an upright stance) can mark moments of empowerment. The somatic perspective thus invites Queer individuals to tune in to their felt sense and reclaim their body as a source of strength rather than site of pain.

Complementing this, expressive art therapy provides methods to externalize one's experience through creativity in visual art, dance/movement, music, drama, and writing, all modalities that engage the body and imagination. Expressive arts are both cognitively freeing and somatically engaging; painting, dancing, or drumming involves movement, rhythm, and sensory experience that can bypass purely verbal processing and tap into implicit emotional memories. For Queer individuals, whose true stories may have been suppressed or invalidated, the arts open alternative avenues for self-expression. A client might sculpt clay to represent their guarded heart, or dance to reclaim a sense of sensual joy in their body. Such methods align with Queer theory's challenge to normative narratives; through art, clients can re-author their stories on their terms.

Underpinning both somatic and expressive approaches is Queer theory, which provides a critical understanding of gender, sexuality, and power. Queer theory teaches us that identities are not fixed essences but performed and constructed through cultural norms.[30] It illuminates how heteronormativity and cisnormativity script restrictive roles for individuals, and conversely, how subversive performances (like drag or gender nonconformity) can destabilize those norms. In a therapeutic context, applying Queer theory means questioning any pathologizing or "normalizing" framework that might shame a Queer or trans person's embodied experience. Therapists affirm that there is no one correct way for a body to be or a gender to be lived.[31]

If a non-binary client expresses discomfort with their voice or walk, for example, a Queer-theoretical stance would explore that discomfort considering societal gender norms, not as something inherently wrong with the client, but as a reflection of restrictive cultural narratives. By making these norms visible, clients can more freely choose which aspects of identity feel authentic. Judith Butler famously described gender as a kind of improvised performance. Embracing this idea, therapy can become a rehearsal space for new identity performances. Indeed, some clients may role-play or embody different facets of themselves in session, trying on a more assertive posture or a bolder tone of voice, to "perform" a liberatory narrative and solidify it in their bodily memory. Queer theory thus infuses the process with a liberating permission to play with and redefine the self.

Finally, a harm reduction framework ensures that our approach to liberation remains grounded in compassion, safety, and realism. Harm reduction prioritizes meeting people where they are and supporting incremental change. Applied to Queer trauma healing and body liberation, harm reduction means acknowledging that healing is nonlinear and that individuals need to proceed at their own pace. For many Queer and trans people, harm is an ongoing experience, from daily microaggressions to systemic discrimination. A harm reduction approach validates this reality instead of pressuring clients to "overcome" trauma on society's timetable. It emphasizes safety and autonomy by creating nonjudgmental spaces where clients have control and choice in engaging with therapeutic practices. For example, if a gender-nonconforming client does not yet feel safe doing movement therapy in a group setting, harm reduction would support finding a safer alternative, like one-on-one sessions or at-home practice, rather than forcing exposure. Key harm reduction strategies in therapy include validating the client's lived experiences of harm, collaborating on client-directed goals, and pursuing incremental steps toward liberation. A client's goal might be as modest as practicing one self-compassionate thought per day or attending one Queer community event per month to build social support. Small steps are honored as meaningful progress. Harm reduction also encourages exploring alternative care models beyond traditional medical or psychiatric systems that may have alienated Queer clients.

These theoretical pillars support continuous Queer liberation in therapy and beyond. Somatic theory reminds us that the body is a central theatre of trauma and healing. Expressive arts therapy offers creative, body-engaged methods to rewrite one's story. Queer theory ensures a critical lens on power, encouraging the deconstruction of oppressive norms and the performance of new possibilities. Harm reduction guarantees that our liberatory efforts remain compassionate and client-centered, recognizing the ongoing challenges Queer individuals face. Together, they form an integrative approach in which healing is not just about alleviating symptoms, but about transforming one's relationship to their body and narrative, at a pace that honors personal safety and cultural context. This integrated framework sets the stage for exploring how, in practice, Queer individuals and communities engage in continuous liberation through innovative, affirming, and embodied means.

Liberatory Praxis: Safe Spaces as Experiments in Freedom

If liberation is a continuous process, where does it happen? One answer lies in what we might call liberatory praxis, the creation of intentional spaces and practices where Queer and trans people can experiment with new ways of being. In the context of Queer liberation, "liberatory praxis" refers to communities, gatherings, or therapeutic settings deliberately structured to suspend the usual social rules, allowing participants to test and experience liberatory ways of relating to their body and each other. These spaces function as living laboratories for freedom: pockets of the world where mainstream norms are put on hold, and Queerness in its fullest expression is celebrated. Activists and therapists sometimes refer to such enclaves as temporary autonomous zones, meaning ephemeral spaces where marginalized groups assert autonomy and create new social possibilities. In late twentieth-century New York City, for example, the underground ballroom houses were autonomous zones where Black and Latinx Queer communities vogued, danced, and co-authored narratives of pride. Within these chosen-family structures, participants developed a liberatory identity, freely exploring gender and performance without the constraints of the outside world.

The liberatory praxis element means that such zones are not merely utopian escapes but sites of practice that can inform real-life change. In a therapeutic sense, we can view support groups, arts workshops, or Queer-affirming therapy rooms as laboratories where clients practice embodied liberation. A therapist's office might become a microcosm where a genderqueer client experiments with using their authentic voice or clothing that aligns with their gender identity, with the supportive therapist offering feedback, tools, and a safe container. Clients gain somatic and emotional knowledge that they can carry into the larger world by mindfully performing liberatory acts in these safe micro-environments. This echoes Paulo Freire's notion of praxis of reflection and action upon the world to change it, adapted here to bodily and artistic domains. Each empowering experience in the liberatory space, be it speaking one's preferred name and pronouns and having them respected, dancing with abandon in front of others, or creating art that expresses one's secret truths, serves as a prototype for liberation in the broader social context, inspiring and motivating individuals to continue their journey of self-discovery and acceptance.

A liberatory praxis highlights learning by doing. In traditional talk therapy, a client might intellectually understand that, for example, "There is nothing wrong with my Queer body." But only through experiencing an environment where their Queer body is truly accepted and celebrated can they deeply feel that understanding. Somatic learning requires action and sensation, moving in new ways, feeling new feelings. Thus, these Queer liberatory labs often involve rituals or group practices that engage participants on multiple levels.

Crucially, liberatory praxis is not isolated from the real world; it often carries a political ethos. The existence of a Queer liberatory space is itself a political act of carving out freedom in a hostile environment. During the height of the AIDS crisis, groups like ACT UP not only protested publicly but also formed mutual aid networks and safe meeting spaces where Queer people could connect, grieve, strategize, and support one another. These meetings were laboratories of hope and resistance: The standard rules of silence and stigma around AIDS were stripped away, replaced by candor, anger, and love. Bodies, ill or healthy, were embraced, not shunned. Such environments taught participants that a liberatory way of relating was possible, fueling them to continue fighting for change. In our current era, we see similarly that Queer and trans youth drop-in centers, for example, can have a lifesaving impact. Within their walls, wearing whatever you want, changing your name, or using gender-neutral bathrooms is normalized, experiences that might be impossible at home or school. Clients have described the ballroom scene as having a "lifesaving purpose," noting the foundational lessons about love, care, intention, and affirmation that participants carry. This underscores that what is practiced in these autonomous zones, such as unconditional acceptance and creative expression of self, does not stay only in those spaces; it arms individuals with confidence and knowledge that can be life-sustaining in less supportive contexts.

Liberatory praxis is the fieldwork of liberation. It bridges theory and lived experience by creating zones of free experimentation. Whether in a therapist's office adorned with pride flags and art supplies, a dance floor in an underground club, or a community art studio, these labs allow Queer and trans people to test the hypothesis "What if I am fully myself, and I am safe and celebrated while doing so?" Each time the hypothesis holds, even briefly, it gathers empirical support in the individual's psyche. Over time, the experiments of liberation yield real results: increased self-efficacy, a broadened window of functionality for being seen, and a somatic sense of pride. Continuous liberation relies on these iterative trials, each support group meeting, each drag dress rehearsal, and each collective ritual, contributing to an ever-expanding understanding of what freedom can feel like. Thus, as we turn to specific cultural practices like ballroom, drag, body art, and gender-bending, we will see them as examples of liberatory praxis in action: vibrant arenas where theory (Queer subversion, body positivity) meets practice (dance, performance, adornment) in the service of healing and liberation.

Ballroom Culture and Voguing: Collective Embodiment of Queer Narratives

Ballroom culture events, such as voguing balls, provide Queer and trans people, especially Black and Latinx communities, with a space to physically embody pride and creativity. Participants on the dance floor craft and perform liberatory narratives of identity through dance, fashion, and attitude. The ballroom scene (or ball culture) is a striking example of a community practice that centers the body as a source of liberation. Originating in Harlem in the early twentieth century, and flourishing by the 1960s onward, ballroom was created primarily by Black and Latino Queer folks as an underground subculture of chosen families ("houses") and competitive events ("balls"). Participants "walk," or perform, in various categories, celebrating different gender expressions, fashion styles, or themes, from high glamour to voguing dance battles. Balls are exuberant pageants of identity, where more is more: Participants use elaborate costumes, runway struts, and stylized dance (voguing) to command the space. Underlying the spectacle is a profound purpose. For over a century, the ballroom scene has always been about community, acceptance, and empowerment for those that mainstream society shunned. As one historical account notes, despite evolving trends, the fundamental heart of ballroom, providing belonging and a stage for self-definition, remains intact. In a world that often vilified Queer people of color, the ballroom was a sanctuary where they could not only exist but shine.

Ballroom culture functions as a collective narrative of Queer resistance and joy. Each house (often named after a pioneering figure or luxury fashion house) acts as a family unit, with "mothers" and "fathers" mentoring younger members (their "children"). These roles and kinship terms rewrite the family narrative for those estranged from biological relatives. On the ballroom floor, the stories of these individuals converge. A trans woman walking in the "Femme Queen Realness" category is performing a story: that her womanhood is authentic, that she can claim elegance and respectability equal or beyond that of cisgender women. A gay man voguing in an acrobatic dance battle tells a story, with each dip and pose, of fighting and triumphing over adversity. The audience, which includes fellow Queer folks who understand these subtexts, serves as witness and validator, cheering on the narrative. In therapeutic terms, ballroom can be seen as a giant drama therapy stage or dance therapy studio, where enactment leads to catharsis and integration. Scholarly perspectives have described ballroom spaces as akin to temporary autonomous zones, where conventional societal rules are suspended and new identities enacted. Indeed, a person can change their name, pronouns, and appearance within the ball, and be fully embraced in that role for a night. This fluidity shows participants (and observers) that identity is performative and self-determined, a core insight of Queer theory lived out on the dance floor.

The somatic impact of ballroom participation is significant. Voguing, the signature dance style, is a highly stylized form of movement emphasizing angular poses, swift footwork, spins, and drops. It is an embodied celebration of confidence and flair. Dancers talk about voguing as experiencing a rush of euphoria and release, "letting out" emotions through each sharp movement or graceful flow. Somatically, this can provide relief from the bodily tension of daily vigilance. Many ballroom participants come from backgrounds of trauma, from family rejection, street violence, or simply the chronic stress of racism and homophobia. The hypervigilant nervous system can channel into performance rather than defense on the ballroom floor. The pounding music and communal cheers act like rhythmic auditory stimulation, which can shift one's physiological state. In essence, balls can induce a collective state of somatic resonance: hearts beating to the same music, bodies mirroring each other's fierceness, an atmosphere thick with what some describe as Queer spiritual energy. Research on dance and movement therapy supports the idea that expressive movement in a group can foster deep emotional processing and empowerment. In the ballroom, without it being clinical, similar therapeutic factors emerge; the dance serves as both exorcism (expelling shame and sorrow through sweat and motion) and embodiment (incorporating pride and strength in one's posture and presence). One might say that in voguing, trauma is being re-authored kinetically: Where once a Queer person's body cowered or hid, now it spins and poses boldly in front of hundreds of onlookers.

Ballroom culture also explicitly nurtures intersectional liberation. It arose from the intersection of racism, poverty, and homophobia and directly addresses those layered oppressions. Categories in balls often play on societal archetypes such as "Executive Realness," where Queer people of color dress as corporate business executives, satirizing, and also asserting, their right to inhabit those roles. By doing so, participants highlight the absurdity of exclusionary norms. A Black non-binary youth might win a trophy for portraying a Wall Street banker with flawless authenticity, a powerful rebuke to stereotypes that such spaces are only for white cisgender men.

Meanwhile, categories like "Butch Queen Vogue Femme" allow gay men to express femininity, and trans men or butch lesbians might walk in categories that celebrate masculinity. This fluid movement across gender expressions fights the notion that one must adhere to a single, static identity. As theorist Kimberlé Crenshaw notes, liberation must consider intersecting identities. The ballroom, in practice, has been considering intersectionality long before it was a buzzword: It is a space for Black Queer liberation, addressing both race and Queerness together. By validating the full spectrum of who participants are, ballroom events send an affirming message that directly counters the multifaceted shame many carry. For a Queer person of color who has felt "not enough" in predominantly white

Queer spaces and "too much" in their racial or ethnic community, the ballroom's message is revolutionary: You are perfect as you are, in all your combinations.

From a narrative perspective, we can see how continuous liberation is embodied in ballroom culture. A single ball might last one night, but balls happen regularly, houses meet frequently to practice and bond, and the culture passes knowledge down through generations. It is an ongoing story. Elders of the community teach newcomers how to sew costumes, drop properly without injury, and find their unique style. Oral histories and legends of past ballroom icons are kept alive, creating a lineage of resilience. This intergenerational storytelling is itself healing; as recent research on Queer intergenerational storytelling suggests, sharing narratives across generations provides a developmental resource that fosters resilience and continuity. In the ballroom, the victories and struggles of those who came before become part of the collective narrative, helping younger members see themselves not as isolated misfits but as inheritors of a rich legacy. Every time someone walks a category, they contribute a new chapter to that evolving story of Queer defiance and creativity. Moreover, they carry that narrative when they leave the ballroom and step into the outside world. The confidence gained from one night's performance can help a person "walk" through daily life with more self-assurance. Knowing that a community has seen their beauty and power, they can internalize a counter-voice to society's negativity.

With its vibrant voguing battles, glamorous self-presentation, and house family structure, ballroom culture epitomizes how community expressive arts facilitate Queer body liberation. It transforms dance floors into sanctuaries of self-fashioning where marginalized Queer bodies are idolized instead of stigmatized. Through the collective energy of balls, participants experience bodily liberation, narrative liberation, and social liberation. The ballroom scene shows that liberation must be continuously enacted to be sustained: Each ball reaffirms community bonds and personal pride, fortifying individuals for the challenges beyond. One participant reflected that the scene could have a "lifesaving effect" in teaching love, care, and affirmation. In the continuous journey of Queer liberation, the ballroom is a celebratory rest stop, a place to recharge, rejoice, and remember that Queer bodies are indeed glorious.

Drag Performance and Gender Play: Subversion on Stage

Drag performers and gender-bending artists use costumes, makeup, and personas to play with gender boundaries. Here, drag queens and a gender-nonconforming youth at a Pride event illustrate how drag spaces invite people of all ages to explore creative gender expression, blending artistry with activism. Drag is one of the most well-known Queer art forms, having exploded into mainstream awareness in recent years. At its core, drag performance involves the theatrical portrayal of gender, often with exaggerated femininity or masculinity, for entertainment, satire, or art. Traditionally, a "drag queen" is someone (not necessarily male-identified) who performs femininity, and a "drag king" is someone who performs masculinity. Still, modern drag has expanded to include a vast array of gender play by performers of all identities. Drag has deep roots; there were drag balls in the 1800s. Today, drag shows occur in nightclubs, theaters, and pride parades globally. While often associated with glitter and comedy, drag has profound liberatory potential. It provides a stage on which identity performance becomes explicit and intentional, echoing Judith Butler's argument that all gender is performative. By taking on a drag persona, individuals can reveal truths through illusion, highlighting that if one can construct a self onstage, one can also reconstruct oneself.

The liberating power of drag operates on multiple levels. Individually, performing in drag can be a way to explore facets of one's gender and expression that everyday life might not permit. For example, a Queer man who was socialized never to be feminine might find tremendous freedom in dressing as a drag queen, embracing hyper-feminine glamour and sass. In doing so, he may heal a part of himself shamed in boyhood for wanting to play with makeup or express vulnerability. A transmasculine or non-binary person might do drag as a king to celebrate masculine energy on their terms, free of toxic masculinity. Even the physical sensations of drag can be freeing; the weight of a wig, the pinch of heels, the bold colors of makeup can create a feeling of transformation, often described by performers as "stepping into" a powerful alter ego. This embodied experience can reduce dysphoria for some and enhance what is sometimes called gender euphoria, the joy of feeling one's external presentation align with one's internal identity or creative vision. The literature notes that being able to openly "breathe" as oneself in public is profoundly healing for trans and gender-nonconforming people. Drag offers a venue to "breathe publicly" in a perhaps amplified form, under the stage lights, with an audience's adulation as oxygen.

Culturally, drag is a form of social commentary and subversion. Through humor and parody, drag performers critique gender norms, politics, and culture. A drag queen might impersonate a famous female singer or a political figure, exaggerating traits to make the audience laugh and think. This subversion has a serious edge: As much as it entertains, it questions why society treats gender and sexuality the way it does. For instance, when a bearded drag queen in a glittering gown sings a power ballad, it confronts observers with the arbitrary nature of associating beards with manliness or gowns with women. Historically, drag provided coded commentary on issues like homophobia or misogyny when direct speech was dangerous. In doing so, it has long been aligned with Queer activism. Notably, drag queens were at the forefront of the Stonewall uprising in 1969; figures like Marsha P. Johnson and Sylvia Rivera are often cited as instigators. Their very existence in defiance of the law was an act of liberation. This legacy continues whenever drag is used to raise awareness or funds for Queer causes, or to create Queer joyful visibility in hostile environments.

From a narrative perspective, drag allows the creation of a persona and a story. Many drag artists construct elaborate backstories or characteristics for their character, a form of narrative therapy or role-play. The performer can project parts of themselves into the character, the confidence they lack, or the history they wish they had, and live it out onstage.

It is a bit like rewriting one's life script in the form of a theater. Someone who is shy offstage might, through their drag alter ego, experience what it is like to be brash and celebrated, thus challenging the limiting narrative that they are meant to be invisible. In the therapy world, clinicians have found that acting out scenarios can help clients achieve mastery or closure. Drag is analogous: a kind of self-directed drama therapy where the client and therapist are one, and the stage is the therapeutic space. The audience feedback, applause, laughter, and shouts of encouragement are powerful positive reinforcement, reinforcing the new narrative of worth and power. The embodied experience of a successful performance can linger in memory as evidence against self-doubt.

Drag also fosters a unique community and mentorship, furthering continuous liberation. Just as ballroom has houses, drag has drag families. Often, an experienced performer will take a newcomer under their wing, teaching them makeup, performance skills, and the ethos of drag. This mentorship and chosen family can be life-changing, providing guidance and acceptance that many Queer youths lack. Drag shows and pageants bring together intergenerational Queer crowds; in the dressing rooms, tips and stories are shared. This communal aspect means that individuals doing drag rarely do it in isolation; they are part of a creative community that validates their exploration. It is common to hear drag performers say that drag "saved their life" because it gave them a family and a purpose. Given the high rates of depression and suicide among Queer youth, especially those who are gender-nonconforming, such forms of belonging are indeed potentially lifesaving.

It is worth noting that drag, like other Queer practices, is not without internal challenges or exclusions; but its evolving nature has increasingly embraced diversity, leading to more inclusive drag spaces. In these dialogues, we see continuous liberation at work, the community reflecting on its norms and expanding them. Today it is not unusual to see transgender drag queens/kings, cisgender women performing drag, and non-binary artists whose drag defies the binary entirely. Drag shows might include performers who mix masculine and feminine in the same look or embody fantastical genders. This trend toward gender pluralism in drag reinforces the liberatory message: You can be whoever or whatever you want to be, and you can change that as it suits you.

In terms of somatic and emotional effects, being in drag or attending a drag show can be cathartic. Laughter and exuberance release endorphins and relieve stress. A study on Queer resilience found that artistic expression is a key source of resilience for Queer youth. One can see drag as a prime example of that. The sheer playfulness of drag, playing dress-up, adopting a stage name, taps into the inner child and invites play, which can repair trauma by providing the safety and fun that might have been missing in youth. Performers of all body types use padding, corsets, or reveals to accentuate their bodies creatively. A big part of drag culture is the message that any body can be made into art. This aligns with the body liberation movement's rejection of narrow beauty standards. Drag thus can help individuals overcome body shame: A plus-size Queer person might feel unattractive per mainstream gay culture, but as a drag queen donning a stunning outfit, they can command a room and feel desirable, flipping the script on fatphobia or transphobia. Research on fat acceptance movements shows that joining such subcultures is motivated by a desire for liberation from thinness culture and an embracing of one's body. Drag intersects with this by often celebrating larger-than-life figures and features; the art form is about exaggeration.

Drag performance is far more than campy entertainment; it is a practice of continuous Queer liberation through theatrical embodiment. On stage, under persona, Queer individuals find the freedom to experiment with and affirm who they are. Drag mocks the rigid frameworks of gender and decorum that have harmed Queer people, turning them into sources of creativity and strength. It builds confidence and community and often provides a first taste of unconditional positive regard for one's most flamboyant, "too much" self. Each show or performance can be seen as a mini liberation, reclaiming power over one's image and narrative. Moreover, because drag encourages evolution (today's persona might evolve or completely change tomorrow), it instills the understanding that identity is not static, liberation must be revisited and renewed. Like in a Liberatory Praxis, the drag stage is a place to test the boldest, most authentic version of oneself and receive loud, proud feedback that yes, this too is you, and you are worthy.

Body Modification and Tattooing: Reclaiming the Body as Canvas

Among the avenues of Queer embodiment, body modification stands out as an intimate and literal way to reclaim ownership of one's body. Body modification includes practices like tattooing, piercing, branding, scarification, and surgical alterations. For Queer individuals, whose bodies have often been sites of other people's control or violence (whether through imposed gender norms, nonconsensual medical interventions, or assault), taking deliberate steps to modify the body can be profoundly liberating. It declares, "This body is mine, and I choose how it looks and what story it tells." In this section, we focus particularly on tattooing as a form of expressive body art that has gained recognition for its healing potential after trauma. Tattoos and other modifications serve as a form of embodied narrative, quite literally inscribing one's story, identity, or values onto the skin. Through this artistic process, Queer individuals can transform their relationship with their body, turning a site of pain into a site of art and pride.

The choice to get a tattoo after experiencing trauma or marginalization is not uncommon. A growing body of research and clinical observation suggests that tattooing can indeed have therapeutic qualities for trauma survivors. In the context of Queer trauma, imagine someone who has struggled with body dysphoria or who has been told their body is shameful. Getting a tattoo can mark a turning point: an act of actively creating something using their body rather than passively feeling victimized by it. A tattoo can externalize an inner struggle or victory, making it visible and tangible. For a Queer person, this might mean tattooing a symbol of pride (like a rainbow, or a meaningful quote) over a scar that came from self-harm, thereby reclaiming that patch of skin as a place of beauty and meaning. Some survivors of hate-based violence have tattooed over their scars or injuries, incorporating them into designs that symbolize resilience. The new image does not erase the wound but transforms it, much like the broader Queer project of transforming shame into pride.

Queer symbolism has long been part of tattoo culture. During World War II in particular, certain tattoos or marks were ways to signal Queer identity covertly. For example, the labrys (double-headed axe) was at one time a lesbian feminist symbol; some gay men tattooed the pink triangle (originally a Nazi concentration camp badge for homosexual prisoners) as a reclaimed emblem of "never again" and pride. Today, Queer and trans people may get tattoos that reflect their journeys, such as butterflies for transformation, coordinates of important locations (like Stonewall in New York), or gender symbols modified in creative ways. Each tattoo often comes with a personal narrative: "I got this after I came out," "This one honors a friend I lost," "This one reminds me of my strength." By wearing these narratives on their skin, individuals integrate their Queer identity and history into their body image in a positive way. Their body becomes a canvas of self-expression. In therapy, discussing a client's tattoos (existing or aspirational) can open dialogue about their values, community, and coping. For someone who feels alien in their body, planning a tattoo can be an act of envisioning a future where they feel at home in their skin, literally making their body more home-like by decorating it with meaningful art.

The tattooing process itself can be part of the healing. It involves elements of ritual: choosing an artist (Queer folks often seek out Queer tattoo artists for comfort and understanding), deciding on imagery, the moment of needle-to-skin, and the aftercare. There is physical pain in tattooing, but it is a pain that one chooses and controls, unlike the pain of trauma, which was inflicted and unwanted. Controlled pain can have a cathartic effect. Some trauma survivors describe tattoo sessions as moments when emotional pain converted into physical pain and then released as the tattoo healed. The biological process of healing a tattoo, your body regenerating skin over the ink, can metaphorically stand for psychological healing. Moreover, endorphins released during tattooing can induce a natural high or calm. The tattoo needle, in a sense, writes a new sensory story on the body: Instead of associating touch with harm, the body now associates touch (through a needle) with creation and agency. Biofeedback and body-therapy literature note that engaging bodily sensations mindfully can rewrite trauma responses. In tattooing, the individual is highly mindful of the sensations and breathes through them, often practicing a form of meditative focus that can restore a sense of ownership over their body's reactions.[32]

Tattoos and piercings are also used to alleviate dysphoria or mark transition milestones. For example, some trans people get chest or breast tattoos after top surgery, turning surgical scars into elements of a beautiful design. This can help normalize the new body and celebrate it. Likewise, a non-binary person might get a tattoo that blends traditionally "masculine" and "feminine" motifs, crafting a visual representation of their identity that they can point to and feel seen by, even if society at large often invalidates non-binary identities. By modifying the body, Queer people are also confronting societal narratives about the body. Western culture, historically, has viewed certain body modifications as deviant or low-class, and at times, specifically associated tattooed bodies with criminality or mental instability. Feminist writer Susan Bordo discusses how culture inscribes meanings on bodies and polices them. In that light, when a Queer person proudly displays tattoos or piercings, they are rejecting the pressure to keep their body palatable to the mainstream gaze. They are asserting that their body exists for themself and their community, not for societal approval. This is akin to the fat acceptance movement's ethos of refusing to shrink or hide one's body to fit norms. For example, a Queer Black woman might tattoo imagery that celebrates her African heritage and Queer identity on her arm, openly challenging both the racist narrative that Black bodies are not beautiful and the heterosexist narrative that Queer bodies are shameful. As noted earlier, a person like that faces compounded body oppression. But she fights against all those layers by taking control of the narrative via body art.[33]

Let us consider a tangible example. Suppose a gay man has long struggled with internalized homophobia that made him feel his love is sinful.

After years of personal work, he decides to get a tattoo of a Greek symbol for eros (love) intertwined with the Queer rainbow. The placement is over his heart. In doing so, he symbolically wears his heart on his sleeve (or chest), declaring that love is not shameful but central to who he is. Every morning when he sees that tattoo, it reinforces a narrative of pride and reminds him of the journey from self-hatred to self-acceptance. This daily visual cue can be more potent than occasional affirmations in therapy because it is part of him now. The body has become a storytelling medium. Research by Weststrate on intergenerational storytelling in Queer communities suggests that making personal stories visible contributes to community resilience.[34] Analogously, making one's story visible on one's body can contribute to personal resilience; a tattoo is an ever-present story that one can draw strength from and share with others who inquire about it.

In terms of continuous liberation, body modification is often not a one-off but a series of choices across a lifespan. Many people speak of the "addictive" quality of tattoos; once you start, you want more. This can be interpreted as a quirk and a continual reclaiming process. Each new tattoo or piercing might mark a new chapter: coming out, ending a toxic relationship, surviving a health crisis, or simply entering a new self-defined stage of life. It exemplifies how liberation is ongoing; as one grows and changes, one might adorn their body to reflect that growth. Unlike the idea of achieving a "perfect body" (a static, oppressive notion), the modified body is always a work in progress, much like the self. It teaches flexibility and adaptation: You can change your appearance dramatically and remain or even feel more yourself. This counters the trauma mindset that you are permanently broken or defined by the past. The modified body loudly declares *I define who I am, and I can transform.* In therapy, discussing clients' tattoos can be a doorway into conversations about their transformation and coping strategies.

Body modification and tattooing offer a deeply personal yet often community-linked means of Queer liberation. By choosing what marks to bear, Queer individuals reclaim agency over their body's narrative. Tattoos turn the skin into a canvas where stories of pain can be rewritten as stories of survival, and where identities can be boldly displayed rather than hidden. The process engages both physical sensation and emotional catharsis, integrating mind and body in the healing journey. It confronts societal judgments by asserting a self-designed image. As an evolving practice, it accompanies a person through life's changes, a continuous creative act of becoming. In a liberated narrative, the scars of the past are not erased but traced over with new ink, contextualized as part of a larger picture of pride, resistance, and self-love. As one survivor noted, a tattoo can transform "the unspeakable" into a visible testament of endurance. In the context of Queer bodies, each piercing or tattoo can similarly be seen as a testament: that this body belongs to its owner and carries their truth, artfully, into the world.[35]

Gender Presentation and Bending Norms: Everyday Acts of Embodied Resistance

Not all liberatory practices happen in organized scenes or through permanent body art; much of continuous liberation occurs in the day-to-day choices Queer individuals make about their gender presentation. This includes how one dresses, grooms, styles one's hair, uses makeup (or not), carries one's body, and otherwise presents oneself to the world regarding gender expression. For many Queer people, especially those who are transgender, non-binary, or gender-nonconforming, creatively playing with gendered aspects of appearance, or gender-bending, is both a necessity and an art form. It is necessary in that being authentic often requires deviating from cisnormative expectations. It is an art that involves personal style, innovation, and sometimes blending cultural gender cues in new ways. Every outfit assembled or hairstyle chosen can be an act of micro-liberation, asserting one's true self despite social pressures to conform. Over time, these everyday acts coalesce into a powerful narrative: a living autobiography written in clothing, posture, and pronouns.

Queer fashion and style have a rich historical context. In eras when open identification was dangerous, Queer communities developed their language of fashion. They used specific colors, accessories, or ways of wearing apparel to signal identity. Today, while these signals are widely known, the spirit of creative signaling lives on in how Queer folks often deliberately break fashion rules. A simple example is the notion of a "gender uniform." Society might expect men to wear pants and women dresses; a genderqueer person might wear a combination, or something entirely androgynous, to convey *That binary does not confine me.* Even within the binary, Queer people often play with conventions: a lesbian reclaiming the once-pejorative "tomboy" aesthetic, a gay man proudly wearing nail polish or crop tops that were once taboo for men. These choices are not trivial; they affect one's perception and sometimes pose harassment risks. Thus, choosing to bend gender presentation requires courage and can build resilience. When someone consistently presents genuinely, their comfort in their skin typically increases, which is a protective factor for mental health. This aligns with gender euphoria, where affirming one's gender through expression leads to positive well-being. Each day that a person leaves the house in clothing that aligns with their identity (versus clothing that appeases others) is a day they reinforce the narrative *I honor myself.* Over time, this narrative can significantly counteract years of internalized self-negation.

From a somatic perspective, gender presentation influences how one moves and feels in their body. Consider a trans person who, before coming out, always slouched and tried to hide their body. Post-coming-out, they might start wearing clothes that fit their authentic style and notice themself standing taller or walking more easily. The link between what we wear and how we carry our body is well-documented in psychology. For Queer individuals, wearing the "right" clothes (right for them) can reduce their bodily tension and anxiety. A trans woman who finally wears a dress in public might feel her breathing loosen and her step lighten, a release of the constant stress of hiding.

Therapists sometimes encourage clients to do small experiments with appearance in safe contexts, almost like exposures to authenticity. For example, a gender-questioning client might be assigned to paint their nails at home and observe how it feels, then maybe wear the nail polish to one

Queer-friendly venue, building up their tolerance and joy for authentic presentation. These incremental steps reflect harm reduction, not forcing someone to be "loud and proud" all at once, but gently expanding their comfort zone. The ultimate goal is for clients to present as they wish in most environments without debilitating fear. Each successful step (no matter how small, like someone complimenting their nails) proves that being oneself is not only possible but rewarding.

Every day, gender expression plays a subtle but significant role in shaping one's self-narrative. When one's external presentation aligns with one's internal sense, it creates a more coherent self-story. Instead of living a painful split, being seen as one thing while feeling like another, a person can narratively unify: *I am who I appear to be; there is integrity between my soul and my style.* This congruence is associated with better mental health outcomes for trans people. Conversely, being forced into hiding is associated with higher stress and trauma. Thus, embracing gender-bending in daily life is a continuous healing intervention against minority stress. It also challenges the broader cultural narrative that gender must be binary and static. Every visibly gender-nonconforming person in public is, whether they intend to or not, doing a small quantity of public education and norm-challenging. Over time, this can shift cultural perceptions. Indeed, attitudes have evolved partly because more people have seen gender-diverse individuals in everyday life and realized the sky does not fall. Recall the feminist dictum "the personal is political." A non-binary person's fashion choices at the grocery store might seem personal, but they collectively push political change by expanding what is considered acceptable.

Queer youth often experiment with gender presentation as a way of finding themselves. It is not unusual for a teenager in a Queer community to go through stages, one year goth and androgynous, next year bright rainbow hair and flamboyant, as they test different identities. This experimentation should be seen as a healthy exploration rather than confusion. It is akin to trying different artistic mediums to see which best expresses your vision. Some contemporary movements, like "genderfuck" fashion, explicitly aim to mess with observers' assumptions by mixing signals, such as a full beard with a flowery dress and combat boots. This can be a playful assertion that gender norms are essentially a social game, and Queer people can play it better because they are aware it is a game. The outcome for the individual is often a felt sense of empowerment. If you can walk down the street in an outfit that makes people double-take and you still feel good about yourself, it builds a kind of internal armor. You have proven to yourself that you, not others, define your worth or your style.

For some Queer folks, minimalist or neutral presentation is liberating; not everyone will go toward flamboyance. For instance, an agender person might find freedom in deliberately choosing very neutral clothing to erase gender cues and thus feel seen as just a person. Liberation is about authenticity, not any one look. Intentionality is key: Rather than feeling coerced, the individual chooses how to present. One client in narrative therapy described donating all the dresses she was forced to wear in her youth and replacing her wardrobe with clothes she likes; this act was symbolic of shedding an old narrative and writing a new one. Therapists can encourage clients to use such concrete actions as narrative metaphors, such as cutting one's hair short as cutting away the past or growing it out as allowing oneself to take up space.

We should also mention intersectional factors here. Culture and ethnicity influence gender expression norms, so Queer people of color navigate additional layers. For example, what it means to dress "like a man" or "like a woman" can vary culturally. A Queer South Asian person might wear traditional clothing of a gender they were not assigned at birth as a statement, mixing cultural pride with transition. This can be doubly liberating, reclaiming cultural heritage and gender identity together. Intersectionality reminds us that challenging one norm can sometimes conflict with another; there may be pressure, for instance, within a cultural community not to deviate from traditional gender roles. Thus, when someone does, it is a courageous act of liberation. It might involve negotiating respect for one's culture while insisting on one's truth, a complex narrative that many Queer folks manage with grace, finding ways to honor their roots while being authentic.

Gender presentation is a continual canvas for liberation, much like an ongoing performance art piece where the stage is the world. It requires tuning out external noise and tuning in to the body's desires and comfort. Over time, as one consistently presents in alignment with self, their body is trained to feel safer in authenticity. The initial adrenaline of stepping out as visibly Queer may give way to a calm confidence. One's style might inspire others; seeing a proudly gender-bending person can give peers or younger folks the courage to try it themselves. This is how liberation spreads socially: One person's self-liberation implicitly permits others. The more common diverse gender expression becomes in a community, the more reinforced everyone's liberation is, because each person becomes less of an outlier or target. The clothes, hairstyles, and gestures Queer individuals choose each day are threads in the larger tapestry of liberation narrative. They seem mundane, but they are significant. Through them, Queer people assert control over their image and declare, often without words, *I define myself.* This steady assertion chips away at internalized oppression and gradually normalizes Queer embodiment in society. It is continuous liberation because it is not a single but a daily event, even hourly. Every time one corrects someone on one's pronoun or resists the urge to dress to blend in and instead dresses to be seen, one is practicing liberation. These practices accumulate, building a life that is increasingly congruent and free. In an ultimate sense, living openly in one's Queer body, moving through the world without collapsing oneself, is both the goal and the path of continuous liberation.

Harm Reduction in Community: Safety and Support for Ongoing Liberation

While exploring ballroom, drag, body art, and gender expression, we have seen how liberatory practices enable Queer individuals to flourish. But it is equally important to discuss how to sustain these practices in the face of real-world challenges. This is where the harm reduction philosophy extends from the therapy room into the community and cultural life. Ongoing liberation does not mean being free of all harm; indeed, Queer and trans bodies still contend with external threats (discrimination, violence, stigma) and internal struggles (dysphoria, trauma memories). Therefore, communities often implicitly or explicitly adopt harm reduction strategies to make liberatory spaces as safe and accessible as possible. In this section, we consider how harm reduction principles (meeting people where they are, incremental change, and prioritizing safety and autonomy) manifest in Queer community practices. By doing so, we acknowledge that liberation is not a linear path from oppression to freedom, but a winding road where people may need rest stops, first-aid stations, and companions to travel with. One key aspect is the creation of safer spaces.

In Queer communities, a safer space is an environment intentionally designed to minimize the risk of harassment or trauma and to maximize inclusion. Examples include Queer community centers, Queer youth drop-ins, Pride events, or online forums moderated to enforce respectful conduct. Safer spaces function as communal harm reduction: They recognize the ongoing harm many face in society and carve out zones where that harm is reduced or absent. For instance, a Queer art workshop might have ground rules against body-shaming language and an expectation of using everyone's affirmed names and pronouns, measures that reduce the microaggressions participants might otherwise endure in general art classes. Doing so allows participants to engage in the liberatory act of creativity without looking over their shoulder. In harm reduction terms, this is analogous to providing clean needles and a supervised setting for someone who uses drugs: It does not eliminate the broader issue (society's transphobia, in our analogy), but it provides a context in which the person can pursue well-being with less risk of immediate harm. Many Queer and trans people describe feeling able to breathe in these safer spaces in a way they cannot elsewhere, which is crucial for healing.

Peer support is another harm reduction-oriented element prevalent in Queer communities. Peers with similar identities or experiences can offer validation and practical advice in ways that professionals or family might not. Think of a transgender peer support group: Members share tips on binding or tucking safely, on navigating healthcare, or coping with dysphoria triggers. This sharing of knowledge is harm reduction; advising someone on how to bind their chest without injuring themselves, or how to manage hormone therapy side effects, directly reduces physical harm. It also reduces psychological harm by normalizing experiences (realizing *I am not the only one struggling with this*) and providing hope (*My peer went through this and is doing okay now*). Within the expressive practices we have discussed, peer support is integral: Drag families mentor novices about both performance and personal resilience; ballroom houses provide emotional and sometimes financial support to their members (keeping them off the streets or away from exploitative situations); tattoo communities might exchange information on Queer-friendly, safe studios; fashion and style forums might help a young person figure out how to do a masculine look without expensive surgery. In essence, the community acts as a collective caregiver, embodying the harm reduction idea that people are likelier to thrive when given nonjudgmental support rather than punishment or isolation.

Because incremental participation is encouraged, people can join liberatory activities comfortably. Not everyone is ready to vogue onstage or march in a parade, especially if they are still grappling with fear and trauma. Harm reduction philosophy, applied here, might say: *Any participation is valid, start where you feel safe.* A person might begin by attending a ballroom event as a spectator or experimenting with drag makeup at home before ever considering performing. Communities often have entry-level roles, like being the DJ, helping with costumes, or being a stagehand at a show, so people can get involved without being in the spotlight until they are ready. Respect for individual pacing reflects the principle that transformation is often slow and nonlinear. By allowing individuals to dip a toe in and withdraw if needed, communities prevent the all-or-nothing scenario that might deter people from engaging. Over time, incremental involvement can build one's confidence to take on more prominent, riskier roles if desired.

Another aspect of harm reduction is addressing burnout and providing recovery within these liberatory communities. Activism and performance can be exhausting, and marginalized individuals are prone to burnout from simply navigating life. Recognizing this, many Queer groups emphasize self-care and mutual care. For instance, after intense voguing battles or activism campaigns, there may be healing circles or rest days to process emotions (some ballroom events even end with a cool-down discussion among participants). Harm reduction reminds us that pushing too hard can cause new harm; thus, a sustainable liberation movement ensures people can step back when needed. Some houses in the ballroom will bench a member for a cycle if they notice them struggling with life issues, emphasizing taking care of their health first, a statement that says *it is okay not to be okay and we will support you until you are ready again,* rather than penalizing absence. This aligns with the harm reduction ethic of compassion over punishment.

Inclusive practices also reduce harm by acknowledging intersectionality. We discussed how intersectionality complicates liberation; in practical terms, communities try to minimize harm by including all intersecting identities. For example, ensuring events are accessible to people with disabilities reduces the harm of exclusion. Recognizing the challenges faced by Queer people of color and creating spaces can reduce the harm of racism within Queer contexts. Similarly, sensitivity to economic disparities, such as offering a sliding scale or free entry to those who cannot pay or sharing clothing so those who cannot afford elaborate outfits can still participate, exemplifies reducing the harm of class inequality. Hassan emphasizes that liberatory harm reduction is rooted in community care and social justice.[36] We see this when communities actively work not to replicate oppressive dynamics internally.

In therapeutic or support group settings, harm reduction encourages letting each person decide how much to disclose and in what way, giving them "narrative safety." In expressive communities, this might translate to, for instance, respecting stage personas and not outing a performer's off-stage identity or not prying into the meaning of someone's tattoo unless they volunteer it. Individuals protect themselves from vulnerability, hangovers, or exploitation by controlling their narrative disclosure. Over time, as trust builds, they might share more, but it remains their choice. This resonates with the idea that voice should be invited, not forced, supporting continuous liberation by ensuring each step (or each spoken word) is voluntary and thus empowering, not re-traumatizing.

The principles of harm reduction weave through Queer community liberation practices as the care infrastructure that holds up the expressive freedom. They acknowledge that while we strive for a world without oppression, we are not there yet, so we must skillfully navigate and mitigate the risks. By creating safer spaces, fostering peer support, allowing incremental engagement, promoting inclusivity, and respecting personal limits, Queer communities help individuals persist on the journey of liberation without burning out or being harmed anew. This approach treats liberation not as a reckless leap into the unknown but as a guided path where travelers have support, rest, and resources. In the spirit of "saving our own lives" through liberatory practice, harm reduction in the community ensures that "getting free" does not come at the cost of well-being, but rather in tandem with healing. Continuous liberation is sustainable liberation, an ongoing movement fed by joy and protected by care.

Liberation as an Ever-Evolving Narrative

We have journeyed through the realms of theory and practice to understand how Queer body liberation is continually cultivated. We have seen that liberating the Queer body narrative is not a singular event or technique but a holistic process, one that engages personal healing and community transformation in tandem. It is at once profoundly personal (felt in the sinews, the heartbeat, the private moments of self-acceptance) and inherently political (visible in public art, collective celebrations, and acts of defiance against oppressive norms). By integrating somatic awareness, expressive arts, Queer theory insight, and harm reduction pragmatism, we arrive at a multifaceted approach that honors the full humanity of Queer individuals. In this concluding section, we reflect on the significant themes and envision how this continuous liberation can proceed.

Narrative liberation has been a core theme: the idea that when Queer people can reclaim authorship of their own stories, especially the stories written on their bodies, profound healing occurs. We explored how expressive arts and community rituals allow for re-authoring. The narrative that emerges is one of agency and pride: a shift from feeling like one's life is dictated by trauma and marginalization to feeling like an active creator of meaning and destiny. This does not mean erasing pain but contextualizing it as part of a broader story of survival and triumph. It also means reframing identities from sources of shame to sources of strength. A poignant example we touched on is turning the "victim" narrative into an "activist" or "healer" narrative; many Queer individuals take what hurt them and forge tools to help others (and in doing so, help themselves). This alchemy of narrative is liberation in action. As therapists and allies, supporting this narrative evolution involves deep listening and validation, offering tools of expression, and bearing witness to clients' truths without judgment. In community, it involves platforms for storytelling and remembering (like Queer archives, open mic nights, intergenerational dialogues).

Embodied healing is inseparable from narrative here; the story is told, felt, and enacted. We emphasized that trauma and liberation live in the body. Thus, each liberatory practice has an embodied component: breathing through a movement that once triggered panic, feeling the solid ground under one's feet while standing proudly in front of a crowd, or physically marking one's skin as an assertion of "mine." The therapeutic implication is clear: Talking alone is not enough to heal deep wounds; the body must be involved in therapy for the changes to take root. Somatic interventions, movement therapy, and art-making are not adjuncts but core methods to treat the whole person. Somatics and art give access to what words cannot reach, and allow release where logic fails.

Positive body-based experiences, joy, pleasure, and calm are not luxuries but vital parts of recovery from trauma. It has been observed how expressive acts create new, positive memories that the body can retain. A Queer body that has danced freely in a crowd or felt the loving touch of a comrade gains a reference point of safety and happiness to counterbalance the imprint of violence or rejection. In short, liberatory practice plants seeds of body-felt hope that can flourish with time. Intersectionality and inclusivity ensure that this process truly liberates all Queer bodies, not just a privileged subset. The overarching insight is that liberation is a broad landscape with many paths, and each person may need a slightly different route. What matters is that all routes are heading toward the same horizon of freedom and that travelers respect and aid one another. Intersectionality in practice breeds empathy: a realization that while one aspect of oppression might not affect me, it affects my Queer sibling, and thus their fight is my fight too. In a liberated future, Queer solidarity would mean that gay men stand against transphobia, white Queers against racism, cis Queers against ableism, and so on, because we understand these all intersect in our community. The narrative of liberation then becomes a collective narrative. It is the story of a people, not just persons, a people diverse and vibrant, united by a common quest to live fully and justly.

Creative expression and culture appear as the lifeblood of this collective narrative, and creativity is both the means and the message of liberation. It asserts that Queer communities can imagine and enact alternatives to what exists. Ballroom imagined a world of luxury and fame for Black and Brown Queer folks who were excluded from those realms and made it a reality in their venues. Drag imagines gender as limitless play and makes that real on stage. These creative acts hint at what José Esteban Muñoz called "Queer futurity," glimpses of a utopian potentiality in the present, often seen in performance and art.[37] Every time a Queer person creates something true to themself, they are, in a sense, pulling a piece of that better future into the now. This is perhaps why Queer liberation has such a strong artistic bent: Art allows us to inhabit the future we want, even if briefly, which fuels us to keep going. Thus, the concluding vision is one where art, play, and expression are not by-products of liberation but central pillars. Societies that embrace Queer people will be societies that celebrate difference, creativity, and embodied joy for everyone.

It is essential to acknowledge that liberation is ongoing, with new challenges constantly arising. The sociopolitical landscape can shift, progress in one decade, backlash in another. We see this in modern times, where gains like marriage equality coincided with heightened anti-trans legislation. Continuous liberation means staying adaptable and resilient in such ebb and flow. The practices and principles we discussed are tools for the long haul. They help individuals and communities weather storms by providing internal strength (through healed narratives and bodies) and external care networks. Liberation is thus not a finish line but a way of life, a commitment to ongoing self-reflection, healing, creative action, and solidarity. It asks, as Audre Lorde does, for us to continuously transform silence into language and action. In practical terms, that could mean regularly checking in with oneself ("Am I expressing or suppressing?"), staying engaged in community efforts, and passing on knowledge to the next generation.

We have moved from understanding Queer narratives and harm reduction, through exploring somatics and expressive therapies, to now envisioning how these play out in cultural contexts and can be sustained. The take-home message is one of hope grounded in practice. Liberation is not a naive dream; it is made real daily through intentional acts of courage, creativity, and care. It lives in the support group circles, in the beats of Queer nightclubs, in the brushstrokes of Queer artists, in the quiet breathing exercises of a trans client overcoming a panic attack, and in the chants of protestors demanding justice. Each of these moments is significant; together, they form a powerful movement. As we move forward, clinicians and community members have roles to play. Therapists can continue to integrate these insights, creating therapeutic environments that are affirming, body-aware, creative, and justice-informed. They can see themselves not just as treaters of conditions but as facilitators of liberation, walking alongside clients on a path of growth and self-realization. Community organizers and artists will keep doing what they have done, innovating, supporting, challenging, and collaborating more with healing professionals to bridge gaps between formal therapy and community healing.

The story of continuous liberation is far from over. With each chapter, in books, in lives, that is written with authenticity and courage, we move closer to the world we envision: one where Queer bodies are not just healed from trauma but are sources of wisdom, creativity, and liberation for all. In liberating the narrative, in embodying our truths, we truly *move closer to a world where every body, in all its Queerness and complexity, can tell their story without fear.*

Case Example: Healing Trauma Through Poetry, Queer Sanctuary, and Brave Space

The client is a white genderqueer individual (they/them) assigned female at birth, in their mid-thirties, who presented for therapy after a traumatic online harassment incident. Specifically, the client was doxxed: Their personal identifying information was maliciously exposed on the internet. Doxxing is the nonconsensual public release of private information with the intent to intimidate, shame, or harm the victim. In this case, the doxxing attack was accompanied by transphobic slurs and threats from strangers, leaving the client in a state of fear and crisis. They reported acute post-traumatic stress symptoms: hypervigilance, insomnia, anxiety around personal safety, and an intense fear of further victimization. Such reactions are common in doxxing victims. The client also described feeling unsafe expressing their queer identity publicly, which illustrates the silencing impact that doxxing can have on marginalized individuals. These presenting issues, trauma symptoms and identity-related distress, became the initial focus in therapy.

As we explored the client's background, several salient factors emerged. The client had embraced their genderqueer identity in early adulthood, navigating a journey of identity development in the context of a largely cisnormative environment. They recounted past experiences of misgendering and minor harassment, but no prior trauma approached the severity of doxxing. Family support was positive, and the client was in a stable monogamous relationship at the time of therapy. Their partner, also queer, provided a consistent source of emotional support and affirmation. The client noted that this relationship was a lifeline during the doxxing crisis, helping them feel loved and grounded when their sense of safety was shattered. The therapeutic focus, however, remained on the individual client's healing process. Prior to this incident, the client had no significant mental health history and had not engaged in therapy. Thus, therapy began with building trust and understanding the client's multifaceted stressors: the acute trauma of the doxxing and the chronic stress of living as a genderqueer person in an often-hostile social climate.

Therapy was conducted within a client-centered framework. At the outset, I prioritized establishing a physically and emotionally safe environment. This was achieved by clearly conveying respect for the client's gender identity and ensuring the client had control over the pace of therapy. The therapy room itself was framed as an affirming sanctuary where the client would face no judgment or misunderstanding regarding their queer identity. This sense of safety and trust was essential for healing to occur. Moreover, I operated with cultural sensitivity, acknowledging how minority stress, ongoing discrimination, and microaggressions contributed to the client's trauma reactions.

This framing empowered the client to engage in courageous self-reflection. They understood that their feelings of terror and humiliation were valid, and that part of healing would involve bravely processing those feelings rather than continuing to retreat in fear. Throughout treatment, I maintained transparency and collaboration, reinforcing that the client was in control of their healing, a key trauma-informed principle of empowerment and choice.

The overall therapeutic approach integrated elements of narrative therapy and expressive arts therapy alongside more standard trauma-focused techniques. Given the client's creative inclination, I introduced the idea of using poetry as a therapeutic tool early in treatment. This was framed within an affirmative approach: Writing could serve as a means for the client to reclaim their voice and craft their narrative on their terms, counteracting the disempowerment of being doxxed.

In the initial sessions, we focused on reducing acute distress and ensuring the client felt safe both within and outside of the sessions. I worked with the client on basic anxiety management and grounding techniques to help manage their panic symptoms. Together, we created a personalized "safe place imagery" exercise: The client visualized a sanctuary in detail, a comforting, private room filled with symbols of queer pride and safety, to use in moments of overwhelm. This internal Queer sanctuary visualization became a calming ritual for the client, reinforcing that they had a mental refuge no matter how chaotic external events felt.

Additionally, I encouraged the use of real-world queer-friendly spaces. With the client's consent, I provided referrals to a local Queer community center known for its support groups, a real-life queer sanctuary. The client was initially hesitant to join group activities due to their mistrust of strangers following the incident of doxxing. I normalized this hesitancy and did not push for group involvement early on, instead focusing on building one-on-one trust and rapport in therapy.

An early intervention involved providing the client with psychoeducation about trauma and minority stress. I explained how the client's symptoms were common, understandable responses to a life-threatening experience; the threat in this case was indirect and online, but it was still deeply personal and violating. Emphasis was placed on the idea that trauma can result not just from physical harm but from intense psychological terror and violation of safety. I also discussed the concept of minority stress, validating that the client's fear and exhaustion were compounded by living in a society where queer individuals often face harassment. This helped the client externalize the blame; by recognizing that societal prejudice, rather than personal weakness, was a significant source of their distress, they reduced self-criticism. The client reported feeling relieved when I labeled the doxxing as a form of gender-based violence, legitimizing their trauma. They expressed that prior to therapy, they worried clinicians might not "get" how devastating online harassment can be. Knowing that the clinical community recognizes its severity (for example, acknowledging that doxxing aims to instill panic and silence victims) empowered the client to engage more openly in treatment.

As the client's acute anxiety stabilized over several weeks, therapy shifted toward processing the trauma and the client's emotions through expressive writing, particularly poetry. Writing was introduced carefully and in line with the client's readiness. Early on, I encouraged the client to keep a journal to express their feelings between sessions freely. They began journaling about nightmares and fears, which helped externalize some of the ruminations. Building on this, I shared with the client that poetry has historically been a cathartic outlet for Queer individuals facing oppression. They discussed how queer communities have often turned to poetry and spoken word to assert their identities and experiences when other platforms were hostile or unavailable. This context resonated with the client, who had previously found solace in queer slam poetry online.

Over time, I more actively incorporated poetry therapy techniques. In one session, for example, I shared a short poem by a queer author that spoke to resilience in the aftermath of trauma. We read it together and discussed the themes, which helped the client feel less alone in their experience. Next, I encouraged the client to experiment with writing their poetry about their feelings. The client was initially uncertain. "I am not a real poet," they said, but I emphasized that poetic expression is about personal truth, not about formal perfection. Indeed, in therapy, inviting clients to write poetry is a valuable exercise, whether or not they consider themselves poets; it utilizes imagination to foster mental flexibility and helps give voice to emotions. With this encouragement, the client started bringing short poems to sessions. These poems, written in free verse, captured snapshots of their emotional state: anger at the harassers, grief for the loss of anonymity, and determination to survive. Writing in verse allowed the client to condense overwhelming feelings into imagery and words, which made the emotions feel more manageable. This aligns with the literature, which notes that when a client constructs a poem, they engage both the emotional and cognitive parts of the brain, facilitating the integration of the traumatic experience. For this client, seeing their fears and hopes laid out on paper brought a sense of order to internal chaos. It also gave them a voice in a situation where they had felt voiceless, a crucial corrective experience after being silenced by fear.

As therapy progressed, the act of writing poetry evolved from a coping mechanism into a more profound tool for processing. I guided the client in exploring the narratives within their poems. For instance, in one poem the client personified their fear as a shadow that shrinks when exposed to light. In session, the client reflected on what "light" represented; they identified it as community and self-acceptance. This metaphor then informed concrete goals, such as gradually increasing social contact. In another instance, the client wrote a fiery poem addressing their doxxers, which helped safely express outrage and reclaim power in fantasy. We worked together to process this, distinguishing between the emotional truth in the poem and the practical realities of staying safe. Through these discussions, the client found new personal meaning in the trauma: They began to see themselves not purely as a victim, but as a survivor with agency. This meaning-making is a hallmark of recovery. When trauma survivors successfully reframe their painful experiences, it can yield a multitude of mental health benefits and become a source of coping and growth. Indeed, by reconstructing the narrative of what happened, the client started to experience post-traumatic growth, describing new appreciation for their resilience.

In parallel with the poetic work, I reinforced the therapy setting as a queer sanctuary. Each session provided the client with an opportunity to be their whole self without worrying about being judged for their identity. Seemingly small gestures strengthened this sense of sanctuary; for instance, I displayed a small Pride flag and mirrored the client's language around gender. The client reported that this was the one hour a week when they did not have to "hide or explain" their identity, which was itself healing. As trust deepened, the client grew more open about aspects of their life they had initially been guarded about. In one session, they tearfully expressed the shame triggered by the doxxing: *Maybe if I were not so visible about being genderqueer online, this would not have happened.* I helped counteract internalized blame, reiterating that the responsibility for harassment lies with the perpetrators and societal transphobia, not the client's existence. These conversations, held in a sanctuary-like atmosphere, allowed the client to reaffirm the goodness of their identity. They gradually shifted from feeling *I have to hide* to *I deserve to take up space safely.* This attitudinal change was bolstered by connecting with external queer sanctuaries; eventually, the client decided to attend a queer poetry open-mic night at the community center, combining both community and poetry as safe outlets. Although they were anxious, they described the event as profoundly affirming, a room full of queer people celebrating art felt like "coming home," in their words. Experiences like this, supported by therapy, reinforced that spaces of refuge and celebration for queer identities do exist, undermining the doxxers' power to exile the client from community.

As the client stabilized and gained confidence, I gently introduced exposure to their triggers and empowerment exercises (brave space). Since the doxxing, the client had been completely avoiding social media. While this was an understandable protective measure initially, the client felt it was holding them back in both work and social connection. Their job in graphic design involved some online networking, which they had halted, and they missed interacting with supportive friends online. In the therapeutic space, the client and therapist collaboratively designed a stepwise plan to regain a sense of agency online. This included practical safety measures, such as tightening privacy settings and using a pseudonymous account for personal posts, as well as graduated exposure.

First, they logged into accounts with all privacy controls on, and then gradually, and at a pace they could handle, engaged in low-risk online activities. After several months, the client was able to resume using a private social media profile to connect with friends. These achievements significantly reduced their feeling of isolation. I helped process their accompanying anxieties, using cognitive-behavioral techniques to reality-test fears (for example, examining evidence that the same harassers were not still targeting them, and that it was okay to rebuild an online life carefully).

Another "brave" intervention was inviting the client to share one of their poems publicly when they felt ready. The queer open-mic night mentioned earlier served as an opportunity: The client decided to read a short piece about surviving trauma. Standing up in a room of strangers and trusted friends, proclaiming their story in poetic form, was a highly empowering moment. They transformed a memory of humiliation into an experience of triumph. It was the ultimate act of reclaiming their narrative. In therapy the following week, the client processed feelings from that event; they felt nervous on stage but ecstatic afterward, describing a sense of pride they had not felt since before the doxxing. A brave space for authentic expression, with adequate support, helped the client transform a place of prior hurt into one of pride.

Notably, throughout these challenges, I remained attuned to the client's limits. Bravery was never forced; it was always a choice, framed as an invitation to growth with the safety net of support. This balance ensured that the client did not feel re-traumatized by therapeutic exposures but instead felt empowered and in control of their healing journey. After approximately one year of therapy, the client demonstrated significant positive changes across emotional, cognitive, and interpersonal domains. Trauma-related symptoms substantially abated; the client's nightmares and intrusive memories became infrequent, and their general anxiety levels decreased. They reported feeling safer and more confident in daily life. While some hypervigilance persisted (e.g., they still double-check the privacy of their online posts and remain cautious around new people), it was now a manageable level rather than debilitating. The client had developed a personalized toolkit of coping strategies for stress, including mindfulness techniques, the safe sanctuary visualization, and, importantly, writing poetry when overwhelmed, which helped them handle residual anxiety without meltdown.

The client underwent a notable identity restoration and growth. At intake, the doxxing had driven them to question whether being open about their genderqueer identity was "worth it" or too dangerous. By the end of therapy, the client expressed renewed pride in their identity. "I am genderqueer, and I will not apologize for it," they stated, reflecting a reclamation of the self-worth that the harassers had tried to steal. The therapeutic environment of queer sanctuary and the successful experiences in brave spaces (like the open mic reading) allowed the client to integrate the trauma into their life story rather than be defined by it. In psychological terms, the client achieved a degree of post-traumatic growth, finding strength, deeper self-understanding, and even social connection as a result of surviving the ordeal. Writing and sharing poetry were key catalysts in this meaning-making process, as they enabled the client to reframe their narrative. The client's romantic relationship emerged even stronger.

Although the therapy focused on the individual, the supportive presence of their partner throughout undoubtedly bolstered the client's resilience. The client noted that they learned to lean into support rather than isolate when in pain, a significant interpersonal growth for someone whose initial reaction was to "go silent" out of fear. By the end of therapy, the client was more communicative with their partner about their needs and feelings and expressed gratitude for the "solidarity" the relationship provided. This aligns with evidence that social support can buffer trauma and facilitate positive adaptation. The partner was briefly invited to join one celebratory closing session (at the client's request), where I acknowledged the partner's helpful role. This helped the client openly recognize that accepting help is not a sign of weakness but rather a part of the healing process.

By the conclusion of therapy, the client had transitioned from a state of crisis and disempowerment to one of stability, self-acceptance, and empowerment. They articulated that the trauma, while horrific, had led them to discover inner strengths and creative outlets they might not have otherwise explored. In their final session, the client remarked, "I reclaimed my story." They moved from being a victim of someone else's narrative to the author of their own narrative, to embrace their body, their Queerness, and the essence of their beauty.

PRACTICE EXAMPLE

A Grounding Ritual of Body and Image

In a quiet, welcoming space, invite the client to begin by closing their eyes and taking five slow, diaphragmatic breaths, gently scanning their body from the soles of their feet to the crown of their head, and internally naming any areas of tension, warmth, or ease. Then, with eyes open, empower them with the choice of two contrasting art materials, such as a fluid watercolor wash and bold magazine collage pieces, and ask them to translate those felt sensations onto a large sheet of paper in a free, unedited stream of marks and shapes that mirror the rhythm of their breath.

As color and texture accumulate, encourage brief somatic check-ins, placing a hand over the chest or softening the shoulders, to notice any shifts, and let that information guide their next brushstroke or torn paper edge.

When the visual piece feels resonant, have them set down their tools, stand, and allow the emerging forms to inform a short movement exploration, perhaps swaying, reaching, or stepping in time with the artwork. Encourage them to return to the image and write a single word or phrase that surfaced during the process, such as "Grounded," "Release," or "I am here," emphasizing their unique interpretation and autonomy in the process.

Finally, standing before their creation, they take three deep breaths, honoring both the body's wisdom and the narrative they have externalized. This is a seamless somatic and expressive art practice that is accessible to any person, regardless of identity or background, fostering a sense of inclusion and connection.

Notes

CHAPTER 1
QUEER BODIES' NARRATIVES

1 S. Farnfield, review of *Expressive Therapies*, ed. Cathy A. Malchiodi, *British Journal of Social Work* 35, no. 8 (August 15, 2005): 1428–30, https://doi.org/10.1093/bjsw/bch377.

2 Catherine Hyland Moon, *Materials & Media in Art Therapy: Critical Understandings of Diverse Artistic Vocabularies* (Routledge, 2010).

3 Judith Aron Rubin, *Approaches to Art Therapy: Theory and Technique* (Routledge, 2016).

4 Pat Ogden, Clare Pain, and Kekuni Minton, *Trauma and the Body: A Sensorimotor Approach to Psychotherapy* (W. W. Norton, 2006).

5 Ogden, Pain, and Minton, *Trauma and the Body.*

6 Julie Tilsen, *Queering Your Therapy Practice: Queer Theory, Narrative Therapy, and Imagining New Identities* (Routledge, 2022).

7 Rachel Yehuda and Amy Lehrner, "Intergenerational Transmission of Trauma Effects: Putative Role of Epigenetic Mechanisms," *World Psychiatry* 17, no. 3 (September 7, 2018): 243–57, https://doi.org/10.1002/wps.20568.

8 Maura Kelly et al., "Collective Trauma in Queer Communities," *Sexuality & Culture* 24, no. 5 (February 25, 2020): 1522–43, https://doi.org/10.1007/s12119-020-09710-y.

9 Charles J. Gelso and Jonathan J. Mohr, "The Working Alliance and the Transference/Countertransference Relationship: Their Manifestation with Racial/Ethnic and Sexual Orientation Minority Clients and Therapists," *Applied and Preventive Psychology* 10, no. 1 (December 2001): 51–68, https://doi.org/10.1016/s0962-1849(05)80032-0.

10 Laurie K. McCorry, Martin M. Zdanowicz, and Cynthia Y. Gonnella, "The Autonomic Nervous System," in *Essentials of Human Physiology and Pathophysiology*

for Pharmacy and Allied Health (Routledge, 2019), 623–43, https://doi.org/10.4324/9780429260773-14.

11 Ogden, Pain, and Minton, *Trauma and the Body.*

12 Tilsen, *Queering Your Therapy Practice.*

13 Kimberlé Crenshaw, "Mapping the Margins: Intersectionality, Identity Politics, and Violence Against Women of Color," *Stanford Law Review* 43, no. 6 (July 1991): 1241–99, https://doi.org/10.2307/1229039.

14 Ella Ben Hagai and Eileen L. Zurbriggen, *Queer Theory and Psychology* (Springer Cham, 2022), https://doi.org/10.1007/978-3-030-84891-0.

15 Ogden, Pain, and Minton, *Trauma and the Body.*

16 Kai P. Blake-Leibowitz, "'Being Able to Breathe Publicly': Trans and Gender Nonconforming People Healing Through Embodied Activity," in *Advances in Trans Studies*, ed. Austin H. Johnson, Baker A. Rogers, and Tiffany Taylor (Emerald, 2021), 177–92, https://doi.org/10.1108/s1529-212620210000032012.

17 J. Scott Young, Craig S. Cashwell, and Amanda L. Giordano, "Breathwork as a Therapeutic Modality: An Overview for Counselors," *Counseling and Values* 55, no. 1 (October 2010): 113–25, https://doi.org/10.1002/j.2161-007x.2010.tb00025.x.

18 Jeff Maliskey, "The History of Queer Resistance and Student Activism at the University of North Dakota" (PhD diss., University of North Dakota, 2022), https://commons.und.edu/theses/4355; Kirsten Leng, "Magnus Hirschfeld's Meanings: Analysing Biography and the Politics of Representation," *German History* 35, no. 1 (February 15, 2017): 96–116, https://doi.org/10.1093/gerhis/ghw142.

19 Kimber Shelton and Edward A. Delgado-Romero, "Sexual Orientation Microaggressions: The Experience of Lesbian, Gay, Bisexual, and Queer Clients in Psychotherapy," *Psychology of Sexual Orientation and Gender Diversity* 1, no. S (August 2013): 59–70, https://doi.org/10.1037/2329-0382.1.s.59.

20 Tilsen, *Queering Your Therapy Practice.*

21 Heike Bauer, "Burning Sexual Subjects: Books, Homophobia and the Nazi Destruction of the Institute of Sexual Science in Berlin," in *Book Destruction from the Medieval to the Contemporary*, ed. Gill Partington and Adam Smyth (Palgrave Macmillan, 2014), 17–33, https://doi.org/10.1057/9781137367662_2; Fred Chou and Marla J. Buchanan, "Intergenerational Trauma: A Scoping Review of Cross-Cultural Applications from 1999 to 2019," *Canadian Journal of Counselling and Psychotherapy* 55, no. 3 (December 3, 2021): 363–95, https://doi.org/10.47634/cjcp.v55i3.71456.

22 M. Rosenthal, "Intergenerational Trauma: An Embodied Experience," *International Body Psychotherapy Journal* 20, no. 2 (2021): 80–86, https://psycnet.apa.org/record/2022-50419-005.

23 Sophie Isobel et al., "Intergenerational Trauma and Its Relationship to Mental Health Care: A Qualitative Inquiry," *Community Mental Health Journal* 57, no. 4 (August 17, 2020): 631–43, https://doi.org/10.1007/s10597-020-00698-1.

24 Gabrielle Gebel, review of *Queering Your Therapy Practice: Queer Theory, Narrative Therapy, and Imagining New Identities*, by J. Tilsen, *Journal of Marital and Family Therapy* 48, no. 3 (July 2022): 949–50, https://doi.org/10.1111/jmft.12571.

25 Abbe Miller, "The Innovative Essence of the El Duende One-Canvas Method," *Journal of Applied Arts & Health* 14, no. 1 (March 1, 2023): 27–45, https://doi.org/10.1386/jaah_00125_1.

CHAPTER 2
BODY LIBERATION AND HARM REDUCTION

1 Katie Margavio Striley and Sophia Hutchens, "Liberation from Thinness Culture: Motivations for Joining Fat Acceptance Movements," *Fat Studies* 9, no. 3 (February 13, 2020): 296–308, https://doi.org/10.1080/21604851.2020.1723280.

2 Striley and Hutchens, "Liberation from Thinness Culture."

3 Striley and Hutchens, "Liberation from Thinness Culture."

4 Striley and Hutchens, "Liberation from Thinness Culture."

5 Striley and Hutchens, "Liberation from Thinness Culture."

6 Eeva Sointu, "Healing Bodies, Feeling Bodies: Embodiment and Alternative and Complementary Health Practices," *Social Theory & Health* 4, no. 3 (July 25, 2006): 203–20, https://doi.org/10.1057/palgrave.sth.8700071.

7 Diane E. Logan and G. Alan Marlatt, "Harm Reduction Therapy: A Practice-Friendly Review of Research," *Journal of Clinical Psychology* 66, no. 2 (January 4, 2010): 201–14, https://doi.org/10.1002/jclp.20669.

8 Logan and Marlatt, "Harm Reduction Therapy."

9 Shira Hassan, *Saving Our Own Lives: A Liberatory Practice of Harm Reduction* (Haymarket, 2022).

10 Hassan, *Saving Our Own Lives*, 241–61.

11 Marie Kuhfuß et al., "Somatic Experiencing—Effectiveness and Key Factors of a Body-Oriented Trauma Therapy: A Scoping Literature Review," *European Journal of Psychotraumatology* 12, no. 1 (January 2021), https://doi.org/10.1080/20008198.2021.1929023.

12 Kuhfuß et al., "Somatic Experiencing."

13 Susan Bordo, *Unbearable Weight: Feminism, Western Culture, and the Body* (University of California Press, 2023), 215–77.

14 Judith Butler, *Gender Trouble: Feminism and the Subversion of Identity* (Routledge, 1999), 3–91.
15 Kuhfuß et al., "Somatic Experiencing."
16 Pat Ogden and Kekuni Minton. "Somatic Experiencing in Expressive Arts Therapy: Bridging Bodywork and Creativity." *Journal of Bodywork and Movement Therapies* 28 (2022): 100–110.
17 Kuhfuß et al., "Somatic Experiencing."
18 Bordo, *Unbearable Weight.*
19 Butler, *Gender Trouble.*
20 Gebel, review of *Queering Your Therapy Practice.*
21 Bordo, *Unbearable Weight.*
22 Mark Pearson and Helen Wilson, "Using Expressive Arts to Work with Mind, Body and Emotions," *Psychotherapy in Australia* 16, no. 1 (2009): 60–69, https://search.informit.org/doi/10.3316/informit.681041767291365.
23 Patricia Sherwood, "Expressive Artistic Therapies as Mind–Body Medicine," *Body, Movement and Dance in Psychotherapy* 3, no. 2 (September 2008): 81–95, https://doi.org/10.1080/17432970802080040.
24 Pearson and Wilson, "Using Expressive Arts," 60–69.
25 Sherwood, "Mind–Body Medicine."
26 Cathy A. Malchiodi, *Handbook of Expressive Arts Therapy* (Guilford, 2023), 3–100.
27 Malchiodi, *Handbook of Expressive Arts Therapy*, 100–201.
28 Lisa B. Moschini, *Art, Play, and Narrative Therapy: Using Metaphor to Enrich Your Clinical Practice* (Routledge, 2019), 6–67.
29 Kuhfuß et al., "Somatic Experiencing."
30 Malchiodi, *Handbook of Expressive Arts Therapy.*

CHAPTER 3
COMBINING SOMATIC AND EXPRESSIVE ART THERAPIES

1 Patricia Sherwood, "Expressive Artistic Therapies as Mind–Body Medicine," *Body, Movement and Dance in Psychotherapy* 3, no. 2 (September 2008): 81–95, https://doi.org/10.1080/17432970802080040.
2 Jennifer Albright Knash, "Engaging Emotional Regulation and Perceptual/Affective Levels of the Expressive Therapies Continuum," in *Art Therapy as Cumulative Trauma Repair* (Routledge, 2024), 45–48, https://doi.org/10.4324/9781032695228-10.
3 Knash, "Emotional Regulation and Perceptual/Affective Levels."
4 Knash, "Emotional Regulation and Perceptual/Affective Levels."

5 Knash, "Emotional Regulation and Perceptual/Affective Levels."

6 Christina Tremblay, "Body Mapping and Body Scan: Meditation and Art Therapy: Literature Review" (master's thesis, Lesley University, 2022), https://digitalcommons.lesley.edu/expressive_theses/650.

7 Cynthia Kerson, "Biofeedback as a Viable Somatic Modality for Trauma and Related Comorbidities," *International Body Psychotherapy Journal* 18, no. 2 (2019), https://ibpj.org/issues.php?issueid=16; Kuhfuß et al., "Somatic Experiencing."

8 Sharon Chaiklin and Hilda Wengrower, *The Art and Science of Dance/Movement Therapy* (Routledge, 2009), 1–55; Cathy A. Malchiodi, *Trauma and Expressive Arts Therapy: Brain, Body, and Imagination in the Healing Process* (Guilford, 2020): 121–42.

9 Apoorva Shukla et al., "Role of Art Therapy in the Promotion of Mental Health: A Critical Review," *Cureus* 14, no. 8 (August 15, 2022): e28026, https://doi.org/10.7759/cureus.28026.

10 Knash, "Emotional Regulation and Perceptual/Affective Levels."

11 Christine Phang and Lisa D. Hinz, "The Expressive Therapies Continuum Assessment: Addressing Criticism of Art Therapy Assessment," *Art Therapy* (January 31, 2025): 1–9, https://doi.org/10.1080/07421656.2024.2436717.

12 Phang and Hinz, "Expressive Therapies Continuum Assessment."

13 Lisa B. Moschini, *Art, Play, and Narrative Therapy: Using Metaphor to Enrich Your Clinical Practice* (Routledge, 2019), 6–67.

14 Phang and Hinz, "Expressive Therapies Continuum Assessment."

15 Knash, "Emotional Regulation and Perceptual/Affective Levels."

16 Moschini, *Art, Play, and Narrative Therapy*.

17 Carole M. McNamee, "Experiences with Bilateral Art: A Retrospective Study," *Art Therapy* 23, no. 1 (January 2006): 7–13, https://doi.org/10.1080/07421656.2006.10129526.

18 McNamee, "Experiences with Bilateral Art."

19 McNamee, "Experiences with Bilateral Art."

CHAPTER 4
PRACTICING HARM REDUCTION IN SOMATIC AND EXPRESSIVE ART THERAPIES

1 Shira Hassan, *Saving Our Own Lives: A Liberatory Practice of Harm Reduction* (Haymarket, 2022), 10–106.

2 Hassan, *Saving Our Own Lives.*

3 Cathy A. Malchiodi, *Trauma and Expressive Arts Therapy: Brain, Body, and Imagination in the Healing Process* (Guilford, 2020): 121–42.
4 Hassan, *Saving Our Own Lives.*
5 Hassan, *Saving Our Own Lives.*
6 Cathy A. Malchiodi, *Handbook of Expressive Arts Therapy* (Guilford, 2023), 100–250.
7 Malchiodi, *Handbook of Expressive Arts Therapy.*
8 Malchiodi, *Handbook of Expressive Arts Therapy.*
9 Hassan, *Saving Our Own Lives.*

CHAPTER 5
LIBERATING QUEER BODIES THROUGH SOMATIC AND EXPRESSIVE ART THERAPIES

1 Tracy Huerta, "Use of the Creative Arts Therapies and Creative Interventions with Queer Individuals: Speaking Out from Silence, a Literature Review" (master's thesis, Lesley University, 2018), https://digitalcommons.lesley.edu/expressive_theses/83.
2 Huerta, "Use of the Creative Arts Therapies."
3 Ashley Austin et al., "Artistic Expression as a Source of Resilience for Transgender and Gender Diverse Young People," *Journal of LGBT Youth* 20, no. 2 (2022): 301–25, https://doi.org/10.1080/19361653.2021.2009080.
4 Judith Butler, *Gender Trouble: Feminism and the Subversion of Identity* (Routledge, 1990), 3–91.
5 Susan Bordo, *Unbearable Weight: Feminism, Western Culture, and the Body* (University of California Press, 1993), 215–77.
6 Angela Hume, "The Queer Restoration Poetics of Audre Lorde," in *The Cambridge Companion to American Literature and the Environment*, ed. Sarah Ensor and Susan Scott Parrish (Cambridge University Press, 2022), 204–21.
7 Lee Edelman, *No Future: Queer Theory and the Death Drive* (Duke University Press, 2007), 1–111; José Esteban Muñoz, *Cruising Utopia*, 10th anniversary ed. (New York University Press, 2019), 19–96.
8 Resmaa Menakem, *My Grandmother's Hands: Racialized Trauma and the Pathway to Mending Our Hearts and Bodies* (Penguin UK, 2021), 27–129.
9 Menakem, *My Grandmother's Hands.*
10 Huerta, "Use of the Creative Arts Therapies."
11 Bordo, *Unbearable Weight.*

12 Antje Schuhmann, "How to Be Political? Art Activism, Queer Practices and Temporary Autonomous Zones," *Agenda* 28, no. 4 (2014): 94–107, https://doi.org/10.1080/10130950.2014.985469.

13 Kevin M. DeLuca, "Unruly Arguments: The Body Rhetoric of Earth First!, ACT UP, and Queer Nation," *Argumentation and Advocacy* 36, no. 1 (1999): 9–21.

14 Kelly Oliver, "Witnessing and Testimony," *Parallax* 10, no. 1 (2004): 78–87, https://doi.org/10.1080/1353464032000171118.

15 Julie Tilsen, *Queering Your Therapy Practice: Queer Theory, Narrative Therapy, and Imagining New Identities* (Routledge, 2021), 11–117.

16 Tilsen, *Queering Your Therapy Practice.*

17 Butler, *Gender Trouble.*

18 Muñoz, *Cruising Utopia.*

19 Paul C. Briggs, Sage Hayes, and Michael Changaris, "Somatic Experiencing Informed Therapeutic Group for the Care and Treatment of Biopsychosocial Effects upon a Gender Diverse Identity," *Frontiers in Psychiatry* 9 (2018): 294830, https://doi.org/10.3389/fpsyt.2018.00053.

20 Briggs, Hayes, and Changaris, "Somatic Experiencing Informed Therapeutic Group."

21 Mira Cantrick et al., "Embodying Activism: Reconciling Injustice Through Dance/Movement Therapy," *American Journal of Dance Therapy* 40, no. 2 (2018): 191–201, https://doi.org/10.1007/s10465-018-9288-2.

22 Christina Tremblay, "Body Mapping and Body Scan: Meditation and Art Therapy: A Literature Review" (master's thesis, Lesley University, 2022), https://digitalcommons.lesley.edu/expressive_theses/650.

23 Peter A. Levine, Abi Blakeslee, and Joshua Sylvae, "Reintegrating the Fragmentation of the Primitive Self: Discussion of 'Somatic Experiencing,'" *Psychoanalytic Dialogues* 28, no. 5 (2018): 620–28, https://doi.org/10.1080/10481885.2018.1506216.

24 Karen Jones, Victoria Clarke, and Luke Annesley, "'I'm Coming Out,'" *Voices: A World Forum for Music Therapy* 25, no. 1 (2025), https://doi.org/10.15845/voices.v25i1.4218.

25 Apoorva Shukla et al., "Role of Art Therapy in the Promotion of Mental Health: A Critical Review," *Cureus* 14, no. 8 (2022): e28026, https://doi.org/10.7759/cureus.28026.

26 Mark Pearson and Helen Wilson, "Using Expressive Arts to Work with Mind, Body, and Emotions," *Psychotherapy in Australia* 16, no. 1 (2009): 60–69, https://search.informit.org/doi/10.3316/informit.681041767291365.

27 Tsun-wei Lily Hsu, "Online Art Therapy: Reimagining Body, Place, Object, and Relations in the Digital Era" (PhD diss., Goldsmiths, University of London, 2024), https://research.gold.ac.uk/id/eprint/36312.

28 Alex Peuser, "Creative Arts Therapies and the Queer Community: Theory and Practice," *Journal of Music Therapy* 58, no. 3 (2021), https://doi.org/10.1093/jmt/thab004.

29 Mehdi Naïmi, review of *Art in Action: Expressive Arts Therapy and Social Change*, ed. E. G. Levine and S. K. Levine, *Canadian Art Therapy Association Journal* 24, no. 2 (2011): 39, https://doi.org/10.1080/08322473.2011.11415553.

30 Page V. Regan and Elizabeth J. Meyer, "Queer Theory and Heteronormativity," in *Oxford Research Encyclopedia of Education* (Oxford University Press, 2021), https://doi.org/10.1093/acrefore/9780190264093.013.1387.

31 Regan and Meyer, "Queer Theory and Heteronormativity."

32 Shawn Ginwright, *Hope and Healing in Urban Education* (Routledge, 2018), 86–142.

33 Ilan H. Meyer, "Prejudice, Social Stress, and Mental Health in LGB Populations," *Psychological Bulletin* 129, no. 5 (2003): 674–97.

34 Stephen T. Russell and Jessica N. Fish, "Mental Health in LGBT Youth," *Annual Review of Clinical Psychology* 12 (2016): 465–8, https://doi.org/10.1146/annurev-clinpsy-021815-093153.

35 Bessel van der Kolk, *The Body Keeps the Score: Brain, Mind, and Body in the Healing of Trauma* (Penguin, 2014), 32–107.

36 Brené Brown, *Braving the Wilderness* (Random House, 2017), 3–71.

37 Butler, *Gender Trouble*; Audre Lorde, "The Transformation of Silence into Language and Action," in *Sister Outsider: Essays and Speeches* (Crossing, 1984), 40–44.

38 Brian Arao and Kristi Clemens, "From Safe Spaces to Brave Spaces," in *The Art of Effective Facilitation*, ed. L. Landreman (Stylus, 2013), 135–50.

39 Ginwright, *Hope and Healing in Urban Education*.

40 Brown, *Braving the Wilderness*.

41 Dean Spade, *Mutual Aid: Building Solidarity During This Crisis (and the Next)* (Verso, 2020), 45–143.

42 Cathy A. Malchiodi, *Trauma and Expressive Arts Therapy: Brain, Body, and Imagination in the Healing Process* (Guilford, 2020), 121–42.

43 Peter A. Levine, *In an Unspoken Voice* (North Atlantic Books, 2010), 157–347.

44 Marlon M. Bailey, *Butch Queens Up in Pumps: Gender, Performance, and Ballroom Culture in Detroit* (University of Michigan Press, 2011), 29–182.

45 Margot Weiss, *Techniques of Pleasure* (Duke University Press, 2011), 143–233.

46 van der Kolk, *Body Keeps the Score.*
47 Levine, *In an Unspoken Voice.*
48 Malchiodi, *Trauma and Expressive Arts Therapy.*
49 Bailey, *Butch Queens Up in Pumps.*
50 Weiss, *Techniques of Pleasure.*
51 Arao and Clemens, "From Safe Spaces to Brave Spaces."
52 Ginwright, *Hope and Healing in Urban Education.*
53 Ginwright, *Hope and Healing in Urban Education.*
54 Brown, *Braving the Wilderness.*
55 Spade, *Mutual Aid.*
56 Levine, *In an Unspoken Voice.*
57 Malchiodi, *Trauma and Expressive Arts Therapy.*
58 Bailey, *Butch Queens Up in Pumps.*
59 Weiss, *Techniques of Pleasure.*
60 Lorde, "Transformation of Silence."

CHAPTER 6
QUEER BODIES, SOMATIC PRACTICES, AND EXPRESSIVE ARTS IN COMMUNITY AND CULTURE

1 J. Scott Young, Craig S. Cashwell, and Amanda L. Giordano, "Breathwork as a Therapeutic Modality: An Overview for Counselors," *Counseling and Values* 55 (2010): 113–25, https://doi.org/10.1002/j.2161-007X.2010.tb00025.x.
2 Christina Tremblay, "Body Mapping and Body Scan: Meditation and Art Therapy: A Literature Review" (master's thesis, Lesley University, 2022), https://digitalcommons.lesley.edu/expressive_theses/650.
3 Abbe Miller, "The Innovative Essence of the El Duende One-Canvas Method," *Journal of Applied Arts & Health* 14, no. 1 (2023): 27–45, https://doi.org/10.1386/jaah_00125_1.
4 Marie Kuhfuß et al., "Somatic Experiencing—Effectiveness and Key Factors of a Body-Oriented Trauma Therapy: A Scoping Literature Review," *European Journal of Psychotraumatology* 12, no. 1 (2021): 1929023, https://doi.org/10.1080/20008198.2021.1929023.
5 Julie Tilsen, *Queering Your Therapy Practice: Queer Theory, Narrative Therapy, and Imagining New Identities* (Routledge, 2021), 11–117.
6 Kimberlé W. Crenshaw, "Demarginalizing the Intersection of Race and Sex: A Black Feminist Critique of Antidiscrimination Doctrine, Feminist Theory, and Antiracist Politics," in *Living with Contradictions: Controversies in Feminist Social*

Ethics, ed. Alison M. Jaggar (Routledge, 1994): 39–52, https://doi.org/10.4324/9780429499142-5.

7 Maura Kelly et al., "Collective Trauma in Queer Communities," *Sexuality & Culture* 24, no. 5 (2020): 1522–43, https://doi.org/10.1007/s12119-020-09710-y.

8 Nic M. Weststrate, Kit Turner, and Kate C. McLean, "Intergenerational Storytelling as a Developmental Resource in LGBTQ+ Communities," *Journal of Homosexuality* 71, no. 7 (2023): 1626–51, https://doi.org/10.1080/00918369.2023.2202295.

9 Rachel Yehuda and Amy Lehrner, "Intergenerational Transmission of Trauma Effects: Putative Role of Epigenetic Mechanisms," *World Psychiatry* 17, no. 3 (2018): 243–57, https://doi.org/10.1002/wps.20568.

10 M. Rosenthal, "Intergenerational Trauma: An Embodied Experience," *International Body Psychotherapy Journal* 20, no. 2 (2021): 80–86, https://www.ibpj.org/issues.php?issueid=20.

11 Sabrina Strings, *Fearing the Black Body: The Racial Origins of Fat Phobia* (New York University Press, 2019), 15–147.

12 Resmaa Menakem, *My Grandmother's Hands: Racialized Trauma and the Pathway to Mending Our Hearts and Bodies* (Penguin UK, 2021), 27–129.

13 Kimber Shelton and Edward A. Delgado-Romero, "Sexual Orientation Microaggressions: The Experience of Lesbian, Gay, Bisexual, and Queer Clients in Psychotherapy," *Psychology of Sexual Orientation and Gender Diversity* 1, no. S (2013): 59–70, https://doi.org/10.1037/2329-0382.1.s.59.

14 Yehuda and Lehrner, "Intergenerational Transmission of Trauma Effects."

15 Kelly Oliver, "Witnessing and Testimony," *Parallax* 10, no. 1 (2004): 78–87, https://doi.org/10.1080/1353464032000171118.

16 Paulo Freire, *Pedagogy of the Oppressed*, 50th anniversary ed. (Bloomsbury Academic, 2018), 43–125.

17 Antje Schuhmann, "How to Be Political? Art Activism, Queer Practices and Temporary Autonomous Zones," *Agenda* 28, no. 4 (2014): 94–107, https://doi.org/10.1080/10130950.2014.985469.

18 Schuhmann, "How to Be Political?"

19 Tilsen, *Queering Your Therapy Practice*.

20 Kuhfuß et al., "Somatic Experiencing."

21 José Esteban Muñoz, *Cruising Utopia*, 10th anniversary ed. (New York University Press, 2019), 19–131.

22 Cathy A. Malchiodi, *Handbook of Expressive Arts Therapy* (Guilford, 2023), 3–100.

23 Malchiodi, *Handbook of Expressive Arts Therapy*.

24 Bani Malhotra et al., "A Conceptual Framework for a Neurophysiological Basis of Art Therapy for PTSD," *Frontiers in Human Neuroscience* 18 (2024): 1351757, https://doi.org/10.3389/fnhum.2024.1351757.

25 Young, Cashwell, and Giordano, "Breathwork as a Therapeutic Modality."

26 Malchiodi, *Handbook of Expressive Arts Therapy*.

27 Judith Butler, *Gender Trouble: Feminism and the Subversion of Identity* (Routledge, 1990), 3–91.

28 Alex Peuser, "Creative Arts Therapies and the Queer Community: Theory and Practice," *Journal of Music Therapy* 58, no. 3 (2021), https://doi.org/10.1093/jmt/thab004.

29 Kuhfuß et al., "Somatic Experiencing."

30 Butler, *Gender Trouble*.

31 Muñoz, *Cruising Utopia*.

32 Simone Alter-Muri, "The Body as Canvas: Motivations, Meanings, and Therapeutic Implications of Tattoos," *Art Therapy* 37, no. 3 (2019): 139–46, https://doi.org/10.1080/07421656.2019.1679545.

33 Alter-Muri, "Body as Canvas."

34 Weststrate, Turner, and McLean, "Intergenerational Storytelling as a Developmental Resource in LGBTQ+ Communities."

35 Alter-Muri, "Body as Canvas."

36 Hassan, *Saving Our Own Lives*.

37 Muñoz, *Cruising Utopia*.

Bibliography

Alter-Muri, Simone. "The Body as Canvas: Motivations, Meanings, and Therapeutic Implications of Tattoos." *Art Therapy* 37, no. 3 (2019): 139–46. https://doi.org/10.1080/07421656.2019.1679545.

Arao, Brian, and Kristi Clemens. "From Safe Spaces to Brave Spaces." In *The Art of Effective Facilitation*, edited by Lu Landreman, 135–50. Stylus, 2013.

Austin, Ashley, Michael P. Dentato, Joshua Holzworth, et al. "Artistic Expression as a Source of Resilience for Transgender and Gender Diverse Young People." *Journal of LGBT Youth* 20, no. 2 (2022): 301–25. https://doi.org/10.1080/19361653.2021.2009080.

Bailey, Marlon M. *Butch Queens Up in Pumps: Gender, Performance, and Ballroom Culture in Detroit*. University of Michigan Press, 2011.

Bauer, Heike. "Burning Sexual Subjects: Books, Homophobia and the Nazi Destruction of the Institute of Sexual Science in Berlin." In *Book Destruction from the Medieval to the Contemporary*, edited by Gill Partington and Adam Smyth, 17–33. Springer, 2014. https://doi.org/10.1057/9781137367662_2.

Ben Hagai, Ella, and Eileen L. Zurbriggen. *Queer Theory and Psychology*. Springer, 2022. https://doi.org/10.1007/978-3-030-84891-0.

Blake-Leibowitz, Kai P. "'Being Able to Breathe Publicly': Trans and Gender Nonconforming People Healing Through Embodied Activity." In *Advances in Trans Studies*, edited by Austin H. Johnson, Baker A. Rogers, and Tiffany Taylor, 177–92. Emerald, 2021. https://doi.org/10.1108/s1529-212620210000032012.

Bordo, Susan. *Unbearable Weight: Feminism, Western Culture, and the Body*. University of California Press, 1993.

Briggs, Paul C., Sage Hayes, and Michael Changaris. "Somatic Experiencing Informed Therapeutic Group for the Care and Treatment of Biopsychosocial Effects upon a Gender Diverse Identity." *Frontiers in Psychiatry* 9 (2018): 294830. https://doi.org/10.3389/fpsyt.2018.00053.

Brown, Brené. *Braving the Wilderness*. Random House, 2017.

Butler, Judith. *Gender Trouble: Feminism and the Subversion of Identity*. Routledge, 1990.

Cantrick, Mira, Terra Anderson, Lucia B. Leighton, and M. Warning. "Embodying Activism: Reconciling Injustice Through Dance/Movement Therapy." *American Journal of Dance Therapy* 40, no. 2 (2018): 191–201. https://doi.org/10.1007/s10465-018-9288-2.

Chaiklin, Sharon, and Hilda Wengrower. *The Art and Science of Dance/Movement Therapy*. Routledge, 2009.

Chou, Fred, and Marla J. Buchanan. "Intergenerational Trauma: A Scoping Review of Cross-Cultural Applications from 1999 to 2019." *Canadian Journal of Counselling and Psychotherapy* 55, no. 3 (December 3, 2021): 363–95. https://doi.org/10.47634/cjcp.v55i3.71456.

Crenshaw, Kimberlé. "Mapping the Margins: Intersectionality, Identity Politics, and Violence Against Women of Color." *Stanford Law Review* 43, no. 6 (July 1991): 12–41. https://doi.org/10.2307/1229039.

Crenshaw, Kimberlé W. "Demarginalizing the Intersection of Race and Sex: A Black Feminist Critique of Antidiscrimination Doctrine, Feminist Theory, and Antiracist Politics." In *Living with Contradictions: Controversies in Feminist Social Ethics*, edited by Alison M. Jaggar, 39–52. Routledge, 1994. https://doi.org/10.4324/9780429499142-5.

DeLuca, Kevin M. "Unruly Arguments: The Body Rhetoric of Earth First!, ACT UP, and Queer Nation." *Argumentation and Advocacy* 36, no. 1 (1999): 9–21.

Edelman, Lee. *No Future: Queer Theory and the Death Drive*. Duke University Press, 2007.

Farnfield, S. Review of *Expressive Therapies*, edited by Cathy A. Malchiodi. *British Journal of Social Work* 35, no. 8 (August 15, 2005): 1428–30. https://doi.org/10.1093/bjsw/bch377.

Freire, Paulo. *Pedagogy of the Oppressed*, 50th anniversary edition. Bloomsbury Academic, 2018.

Gebel, Gabrielle. Review of *Queering Your Therapy Practice* by Julie Tilsen. *Journal of Marital and Family Therapy* 48, no. 3 (July 2022): 949–50. https://doi.org/10.1111/jmft.12571.

Gelso, Charles J., and Jonathan J. Mohr. "The Working Alliance and the Transference/Countertransference Relationship: Their Manifestation with Racial/Ethnic and Sexual Orientation Minority Clients and Therapists." *Applied and Preventive Psychology* 10, no. 1 (December 2001): 51–68. https://doi.org/10.1016/s0962-1849(05)80032-0.

Ginwright, Shawn. *Hope and Healing in Urban Education*. Routledge, 2018.

Hassan, Shira. *Saving Our Own Lives: A Liberatory Practice of Harm Reduction.* Haymarket, 2022.

Hsu, Tsun-wei Lily. "Online Art Therapy: Reimagining Body, Place, Object, and Relations in the Digital Era." PhD diss., Goldsmiths, University of London, 2024. https://research.gold.ac.uk/id/eprint/36312.

Huerta, Tracy. "Use of the Creative Arts Therapies and Creative Interventions with Queer Individuals: Speaking Out from Silence, a Literature Review." Master's thesis, Lesley University, 2018. https://digitalcommons.lesley.edu/expressive_theses/83.

Hume, Angela. "The Queer Restoration Poetics of Audre Lorde." In *The Cambridge Companion to American Literature and the Environment,* edited by Sarah Ensor and Susan Scott Parrish. Cambridge University Press, 2022.

Isobel, Sophie, Andrea McCloughen, Melinda Goodyear, and Kim Foster. "Intergenerational Trauma and Its Relationship to Mental Health Care: A Qualitative Inquiry." *Community Mental Health Journal* 57, no. 4 (August 17, 2020): 631–43. https://doi.org/10.1007/s10597-020-00698-1.

Jones, Karen, Victoria Clarke, and Luke Annesley. "'I'm Coming Out.'" *Voices: A World Forum for Music Therapy* 25, no. 1 (2025). https://doi.org/10.15845/voices.v25i1.4218.

Kelly, Maura, Amy Lubitow, Matthew Town, and Amanda Mercier. "Collective Trauma in Queer Communities." *Sexuality & Culture* 24, no. 5 (February 25, 2020): 1522–43. https://doi.org/10.1007/s12119-020-09710-y.

Kerson, Cynthia. "Biofeedback as a Viable Somatic Modality for Trauma and Related Comorbidities: A New Methodology." *International Body Psychotherapy Journal* 18, no. 2 (Fall/Winter 2019/20): 196–207. https://ibpj.org/issues.php?issueid=16.

Knash, Jennifer Albright. "Engaging Emotional Regulation and Perceptual/Affective Levels of the Expressive Therapies Continuum." In *Art Therapy as Cumulative Trauma Repair,* 45–48. Routledge, 2024. https://doi.org/10.4324/9781032695228-10.

Kuhfuß, Marie, Tobias Maldei, Andreas Hetmanek, and Nicola Baumann. "Somatic Experiencing—Effectiveness and Key Factors of a Body-Oriented Trauma Therapy: A Scoping Literature Review." *European Journal of Psychotraumatology* 12, no. 1 (January 2021). https://doi.org/10.1080/20008198.2021.1929023.

Leng, Kirsten. "Magnus Hirschfeld's Meanings: Analysing Biography and the Politics of Representation." *German History* 35, no. 1 (February 15, 2017): 96–116. https://doi.org/10.1093/gerhis/ghw142.

Levine, Peter A. *In an Unspoken Voice.* North Atlantic Books, 2010.

Levine, Peter A., Abi Blakeslee, and Joshua Sylvae. "Reintegrating the Fragmentation of the Primitive Self: Discussion of 'Somatic Experiencing.'" *Psychoanalytic*

Dialogues 28, no. 5 (2018): 620–28. https://doi.org/10.1080/10481885.2018.1506216.

Logan, Diane E., and G. Alan Marlatt. "Harm Reduction Therapy: A Practice-Friendly Review of Research." *Journal of Clinical Psychology* 66, no. 2 (January 4, 2010): 201–214. https://doi.org/10.1002/jclp.20669.

Lorde, Audre. *Sister Outsider: Essays and Speeches*. Crossing, 1984.

Lu, Liang, and Fiona Yuen. "Journey Women: Art Therapy in a Decolonizing Framework of Practice." *The Arts in Psychotherapy* 39 (2012): 192–200. https://doi.org/10.1016/j.aip.2011.12.00.

Malchiodi, Cathy A. *Trauma and Expressive Arts Therapy: Brain, Body, and Imagination in the Healing Process*. Guilford, 2020.

Malchiodi, Cathy A. *Handbook of Expressive Arts Therapy*. Guilford, 2023.

Maliskey, Jeff, "The History of Queer Resistance and Student Activism at the University of North Dakota." PhD diss., University of North Dakota, 2022. https://commons.und.edu/theses/4355.

McCorry, Laurie K., Martin M. Zdanowicz, and Cynthia Y. Gonnella. "The Autonomic Nervous System." In *Essentials of Human Physiology and Pathophysiology for Pharmacy and Allied Health*, 623–43. Routledge, 2021. https://doi.org/10.4324/9780429260773.

McNamee, Carole M. "Experiences with Bilateral Art: A Retrospective Study." *Art Therapy* 23, no. 1 (January 2006): 7–13. https://doi.org/10.1080/07421656.2006.10129526.

Menakem, Resmaa. *My Grandmother's Hands: Racialized Trauma and the Pathway to Mending Our Hearts and Bodies*. Penguin UK, 2021.

Meyer, Ilan H. "Prejudice, Social Stress, and Mental Health in LGB Populations." *Psychological Bulletin* 129, no. 5 (2003): 674–97. https://doi.org/10.1037/0033-2909.129.5.674.

Miller, Abbe. "The Innovative Essence of the El Duende One-Canvas Method." *Journal of Applied Arts & Health* 14, no. 1 (March 1, 2023): 27–45. https://doi.org/10.1386/jaah_00125_1.

Moon, Catherine Hyland. *Materials & Media in Art Therapy: Critical Understandings of Diverse Artistic Vocabularies*. Routledge, 2010.

Moschini, Lisa B. *Art, Play, and Narrative Therapy: Using Metaphor to Enrich Your Clinical Practice*. Routledge, 2019.

Muñoz, José Esteban. *Cruising Utopia*, 10th anniversary edition. New York University Press, 2019.

O'Connor, James. *Culture Is Not an Industry: Reclaiming Art and Culture for the Common Good*. Manchester University Press, 2024.

Ogden, Pat, Clare Pain, and Kekuni Minton. *Trauma and the Body: A Sensorimotor Approach to Psychotherapy*. W. W. Norton, 2006.

Oliver, Kelly. "Witnessing and Testimony." *Parallax* 10, no. 1 (2004): 78–87. https://doi.org/10.1080/1353464032000171118.

Pearson, Mark, and Helen Wilson. "Using Expressive Arts to Work with Mind, Body, and Emotions." *Psychotherapy in Australia* 16, no. 1 (2009): 60–69. https://search.informit.org/doi/10.3316/informit.681041767291365.

Peuser, Alex. "Creative Arts Therapies and the Queer Community: Theory and Practice." *Journal of Music Therapy* 58, no. 3 (2021). https://doi.org/10.1093/jmt/thab004.

Phang, Christine, and Lisa D. Hinz. "The Expressive Therapies Continuum Assessment: Addressing Criticism of Art Therapy Assessment." *Art Therapy* (January 31, 2025): 1–9. https://doi.org/10.1080/07421656.2024.2436717.

Regan, Page V., and Elizabeth J. Meyer. "Queer Theory and Heteronormativity." In *Oxford Research Encyclopedia of Education* (Oxford, 2021). https://doi.org/10.1093/acrefore/9780190264093.013.1387.

Rosenthal, M. "Intergenerational Trauma: An Embodied Experience." *International Body Psychotherapy Journal* 20, no. 2 (2021): 80–86. https://www.ibpj.org/issues.php?issueid=20.

Rubin, Judith Aron. *Approaches to Art Therapy: Theory and Technique*. Routledge, 2016.

Schuhmann, Antje. "How to Be Political? Art Activism, Queer Practices and Temporary Autonomous Zones." *Agenda* 28, no. 4 (2014): 94–107. https://doi.org/10.1080/10130950.2014.985469.

Shelton, Kimber, and Edward A. Delgado-Romero. "Sexual Orientation Microaggressions: The Experience of Lesbian, Gay, Bisexual, and Queer Clients in Psychotherapy." *Psychology of Sexual Orientation and Gender Diversity* 1, no. S (August 2013): 59–70. https://doi.org/10.1037/2329-0382.1.s.59.

Sherwood, Patricia. "Expressive Artistic Therapies as Mind–Body Medicine." *Body, Movement and Dance in Psychotherapy* 3, no. 2 (September 2008): 81–95. https://doi.org/10.1080/17432970802080040.

Shukla, Apoorva, Sonali G. Choudhari, Abhay M. Gaidhane, and Zahiruddin Quazi Syed. "Role of Art Therapy in the Promotion of Mental Health: A Critical Review." *Cureus* 14, no. 8 (August 15, 2022): e28026. https://doi.org/10.7759/cureus.28026.

Sointu, Eeva. "Healing Bodies, Feeling Bodies: Embodiment and Alternative and Complementary Health Practices." *Social Theory & Health* 4, no. 3 (July 25, 2006): 203–20. https://doi.org/10.1057/palgrave.sth.8700071.

Spade, Dean. *Mutual Aid: Building Solidarity During This Crisis (and the Next)*. Verso, 2020.

Striley, Katie Margavio, and Sophia Hutchens. "Liberation from Thinness Culture: Motivations for Joining Fat Acceptance Movements." *Fat Studies* 9, no. 3 (February 13, 2020): 296–308. https://doi.org/10.1080/21604851.2020.1723280.

Strings, Sabrina. *Fearing the Black Body: The Racial Origins of Fat Phobia*. New York University Press, 2019.

Tilsen, Julie. *Queering Your Therapy Practice: Queer Theory, Narrative Therapy, and Imagining New Identities*. Routledge, 2022.

Tremblay, Christina. "Body Mapping and Body Scan: Meditation and Art Therapy: A Literature Review." Master's thesis, Lesley University, 2022. https://digitalcommons.lesley.edu/expressive_theses/650.

van der Kolk, Bessel. *The Body Keeps the Score: Brain, Mind, and Body in the Healing of Trauma*. Penguin, 2014.

Weiss, Margot. *Techniques of Pleasure: BDSM and the Circuits of Sexuality*. Duke University Press, 2011.

Weststrate, Nic M., Kit Turner, and Kate C. McLean. "Intergenerational Storytelling as a Developmental Resource in LGBTQ+ Communities." *Journal of Homosexuality* 71, no. 7 (2023): 1626–51. https://doi.org/10.1080/00918369.2023.2202295.

Yehuda, Rachel, and Amy Lehrner. "Intergenerational Transmission of Trauma Effects: Putative Role of Epigenetic Mechanisms." *World Psychiatry* 17, no. 3 (September 7, 2018): 243–57. https://doi.org/10.1002/wps.20568.

Young, J. Scott, Craig S. Cashwell, and Amanda L. Giordano. "Breathwork as a Therapeutic Modality: An Overview for Counselors." *Counseling and Values* 55, no. 1 (October 2010): 113–25. https://doi.org/10.1002/j.2161-007x.2010.tb00025.x.

Index

C

D

G

H

J

K

L

M

N

Q

U

V

About the Author

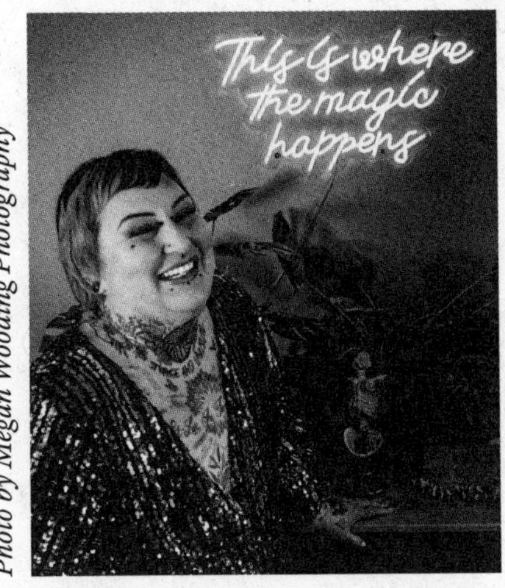

Photo by Megan Wooding Photography

Wednesdae Reim Ifrach, REAT, ATR-BC, ATCS, LPC, NCC, CLAT, is a trans/non-binary art therapist and counselor dedicated to providing gender-affirming, trauma-informed care that emphasizes healing-centered engagement, body justice, intersectional social justice, and equitable access to eating disorder treatment. They co-own and operate Rainbow Recovery, offering clinical supervision, consultations, trainings, workshops, counseling, and art therapy services to clients in Connecticut and Pennsylvania. As a full-time professor at Moravian University, Wednesdae teaches mental health counseling, social work, and expressive art courses, inspiring future professionals. Over the past decade, they have led trainings and workshops for the American Art Therapy Association, National Alliance for Eating Disorders, and Yale University, among others. Previously, Wednesdae founded the country's first 2sLGBTQIA+ eating disorder program, served on Project HEAL's board, and presided over the Connecticut Art Therapy Association. They currently co-chair the Health Professionals in Training Program on the GLMA board. Their expertise addresses LGBTQ+ concerns and trauma, honoring each client's identity.

About North Atlantic Books

North Atlantic Books (NAB) is an independent, nonprofit publisher committed to a bold exploration of the relationships between mind, body, spirit, and nature. Founded in 1974, NAB aims to nurture a holistic view of the arts, sciences, humanities, and healing. To make a donation or to learn more about our books, authors, events, and newsletter, please visit www.northatlanticbooks.com.